how
atmospheric conditions
affect your health

how
atmospheric
affec

TRANSLATED BY *JOYCE E. CLEMOW*

conditions
your health

Michel Gauquelin

𝔰𝔡

STEIN AND DAY/*Publishers*/New York

ACKNOWLEDGMENTS

I wish to express my sincere gratitude to all the eminent specialists who so kindly assisted me with their advice, and in particular to Dr. Jean Rivolier, affiliated with the Center for Allergic Research at Rothschild Hospital; to Valéry Mironovitch, consulting engineer for the Central Society of Meteorological Studies and Applications; to Prof. Giorgio Piccardi, Director of the Institute of Physical Chemistry at the University of Florence; to Dr. Jean Sutter, departmental manager at the National Institute of Demographic Studies; to Frank A. Brown, Morrison professor of biology at Northwestern University, Evanston, Illinois; and to Dr. S. W. Tromp, Director of the Center for Bioclimatological Research in Leyden. I should also like to thank all those who participated in the Fourth International Biometeorological Conference and were interested in my work (Rutgers University, New Brunswick, New Jersey, August 26–September 2, 1966).

CONTENTS

how
atmospheric conditions
affect your health

INTRODUCTION

Since time immemorial, wrote Dr. V. Raymond, men have believed that diseases were associated with meteors,* and consequently that deaths were controlled by these phenomena. They originally thought that the atmosphere was the most influential factor in this respect and was therefore responsible for a great number of illnesses. Then, as knowledge increased, heredity and in particular bacteria took precedence as factors. The truth lies somewhere in between. Diseases due to heredity and bacteria do exist, but so do illnesses resulting from atmospheric phenomena. However, what complicates matters is that often each of these three factors contributes to many diseases.[1]

The relationship between our health and atmospheric conditions has a long history in which legend is interwoven with reality. Hippocrates, the father of medicine, wrote in detail about the atmosphere's influence in his famous treatise "On Airs, Waters and Places." He mentioned all the essential points of the close bonds linking man and the weather. Twenty-five centuries have passed and medicine has earned

---

* The word meteor is derived from the Greek *meteōron* (any phenomenon in the atmosphere). Webster defines the word meteor as any phenomenon occurring in the atmosphere (fog, rain, storms, etc.).

1. *La Presse Médicale* (February 18, 1961).

countless laurels, but for a long time the study of health and the weather has been overlooked and neglected. Two scientific giants, Pasteur and Mendel, were unintentionally responsible for this. The discovery that illness could be due to either bacteria or heredity relegated the study of the weather's effects on our health to second place. However, disasters caused by sudden meteorological changes continued to take their toll together with the other scourges of nature. All of us, healthy or sick, young or old, are affected by these meteorological caprices. I wonder if we are aware of this. If we read in the newspaper that a greenish fog has covered London and caused the deaths of several thousand people, we think that an exceptional phenomenon has occurred. The sudden fear that it arouses in us disappears as quickly as it came, and we soon forget about it. This is a serious mistake: atmospheric phenomena are causing deaths day after day, in both cities and the country.

For several decades medical science has intensified research on the atmosphere to make up for lost time. But many things had to be done: devise measuring instruments; accumulate data; formulate new theories. In some fields, that of air pollution, for example, it was almost too late. But William Petersen in the United States, B. de Rudder in Germany, Sollo W. Tromp in Holland, Giorgio Piccardi in Italy, Jean Rivolier and Valéry Mironovitch in France, and many other investigators were confident. They predicted, confirmed, and partially mastered the effects of most of the factors involved in atmospheric changes that disturb our systems.

The aim of this book is to review their discoveries. I shall analyze the influence of the weather, the seasons, climate, and cosmic forces on our health.

First I shall consider the effects of what is called, for want of a better term, "the weather." This word embodies a large number of meteorological variables. How do they work? Dr. Rivolier wrote, "In medicine, we are very familiar with those nights when all the cardiologists of a city are on the alert because their patients are experiencing acute cardiac decompensations and many myocardial infarctions occur. Hospital wards were sometimes confronted with an alarming situation, especially before the advent of anticoagulant drugs, namely a sudden increase in the number of cases of phlebitis and pulmonary emboli in women who had recently given birth. Nor will any surgeon dispute the fact that on some days all the patients who have undergone surgery have hemorrhagic complications. Why? And why do some of these pathological phenomena suddenly stop for no apparent reason?" [2]

For a long time one of medicine's greatest mysteries was the belief that "the weather" was responsible for disasters occurring in groups. Today it can be proved. Doctors and meteorologists can explain the influence of lethal fogs, devastating winds, sudden drops of barometric pressure, and electrical disturbances in the air.

About thirty-five years ago meteorologists defined the idea of a "front," which is an extremely important notion as far as our health is concerned; deaths occur more frequently while fronts are passing over. I shall examine the reason for this.

As a background to the weather, which varies essentially from one day to the next, there is the majestic rhythm of the seasons. The earth's continual journey around the sun assures their annual procession: spring—summer—autumn—winter. We associate certain pleasures of living with every season: winter sports, walks on the first fine days of spring, seaside vacations in summer; and hunting in autumn. But the seasons are responsible for an entirely different aspect of our physical health and our mental balance. Each season brings its own threat of disease and death. Is it true that the suicide rate is much higher in spring? Why does poliomyelitis strike during the summer, and why are myocardial in-

2. Jean Rivolier, "La Biométéorologie," *Diagrammes* (1965), p. 5.

farctions more frequent in winter? I shall try to answer these and other questions.

The season changes every three months, but the influence of climate is continuous. Its power is so strong that over the generations it has been able to mold man's physical constitution, alter the color of his skin, and influence his psychological state. Some climates are favorable to health, while others appear detrimental. "Just as there are unexplained pathological coincidences, so the therapeutic value of certain places has been recognized. But when it is said that a given area helps certain patients, that is almost all that is said. There is no explanation of why or how that environment is favorable." [3] Is it the temperature, the amount of sunshine, the water, or the fauna and flora that give a place its climatic qualities? Or does its beneficial role reside in the composition of the soil? I shall discuss the latest answers given us by the experts.

One final mystery remains to be solved, more difficult perhaps than the preceding ones—namely, the effect of cosmic influences on our health. In the past, they were considered a part of atmospheric conditions. Then they were exploited by astrologers and charlatans. Still there were such questions as, Why does the moon have the reputation of influencing mentally unstable people, causing women to menstruate, and determining a child's sex? Today these questions are being studied in a modern light. Now with the advent of interplanetary exploration they have a renewed importance. I shall also discuss the role, long unsuspected, of solar and cosmic radiations that penetrate the protective screen of the terrestrial atmosphere and act on our fragile systems.

Biometeorological medicine is a young science. It is developing rapidly because of close collaboration between doctors and meteorologists, and among astronomers, geologists, urban specialists, statisticians, sociologists, and psychologists

3. *Ibid.*, p. 6.

too. It is through teamwork like this that a better understanding of atmospheric conditions has been achieved and that preventive measures based on new therapeutic procedures can be contemplated.

Hippocrates' advice is being heeded: "Through these considerations and by learning the weather beforehand, the doctor will have available full knowledge to help him in each specific case. He will know best how to protect health, and he will practice the art of medicine with success."

CAPRICES OF THE WEATHER

In December 1930, in the Meuse valley near Liège in Belgium, a fog laden with gas and carbon particles persisted for five days. It brought death to sixty-three people and serious illness to many more. The pollution came from the iron, steel, zinc, and glass industries in the area. But weather conditions brought about the disaster. The boxlike configuration of the Meuse valley and a complete absence of wind caused the air to lie stagnant while killing fog went about its work of destruction.

Another disaster took place at Donora, Pennsylvania, near Pittsburgh, in November 1948, and resulted in nineteen deaths. As in the earlier incident in Belgium, the topography at Donora was that of an enclosed valley. Toxic products discharged by neighboring factories together with a persistent fog resulted in catastrophe.

But the tragedies at Liège and Donora are minor compared to the one that occurred in London in 1952. On December 5 it seemed to Londoners that the sun would never rise. An exceptionally dense smog hung over that great city and remained for several days. According to official estimates, it claimed more than four thousand victims during the three or four days that it lasted. Dr. P. J. Meade, appointed to make a study of the disaster, stated: "This event must be considered as the most catastrophic of its kind which has ever occurred on Earth."[1] Not until several years later did the British Government dare reveal the full extent of the tragedy. The authorities responsible feared, and rightly so, that Londoners would panic.

British doctors and public health officials joined forces to study the disaster and make recommendations to prevent a recurrence. Fog itself does not threaten human life. It must be heavily polluted and must stagnate for a long time over one area to become harmful. Unfortunately this is what happened on December 5, 1952, when a high-pressure zone covered almost all the south of England for several days without a breath of wind. These atmospheric conditions existed throughout Great Britain, but the disaster struck only at London. Why? Because of the pollution which prevailed over the British capital and from which the countryside was exempt. British experts estimate that the 1952 smog contained several hundred tons of smoke and sulfur dioxide. Dr. Wilkins recorded the daily levels of air pollution and compared them with the mortality rate. The results are worth examining. This graph shows the number of deaths increasing in direct relation to the concentration of smoke and sulfur dioxide.* Dr. Wilkins stated: "Here is indisputable proof of the devastating role of air pollution."

It is important to make a distinction between smog of the sort that brought disaster to London (a mixture of smoke, fog, and sulfur dioxide) and modern photochemical smog. Photochemical smog is a complex mixture of gases and particles manufactured by sunlight out of the raw materials —nitrogen oxides and hydrocarbons—discharged into the atmosphere, chiefly by the automobile. Los Angeles used to be a prime example of this type of smog, but it no longer has a monopoly on it. It is now found in almost every metropolitan area.

1. P. J. Meade, "Smog, Its Origins and Prevention" in S. W. Tromp, ed., *Medical Biometeorology* (New York, 1963), p. 144.

* An oxygen compound (SO_2) derived from sulfur; a colorless, semi-asphyxiating gas.

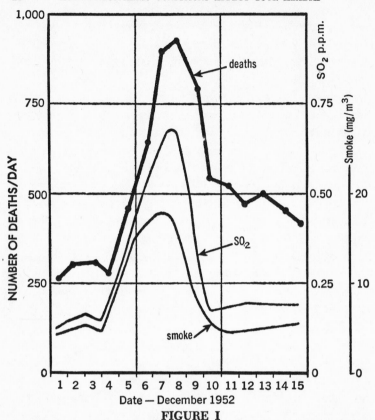

FIGURE I

LONDON SMOG, DECEMBER 5 TO DECEMBER 9, 1952

The increase in the number of deaths is due to an abnormally high concentration of smoke and sulfur dioxide (SO_2) in the atmosphere.[2]

The urban atmosphere in the United States, for instance, is choked with particulates. Los Angeles estimates its aerosol emissions from gasoline-powered vehicles at 40 tons a day. An average winter day in New York produces approximately 335 tons of particulate matter. In the winter of 1963 during a period of high pollution and inversion, more than 400 people in New York died because of air pollution.

2. *Ibid.*, p. 145.

But it is not just the very large cities which have problems. Particulate levels of over 100 micrograms per cubic meter are considered unsatisfactory. Let us look at the situation of these cities as reported by the National Air Pollution Control Administration in 1968:

Charleston, West Virginia	Minimum	43
	Maximum	977
	Average	306
Pittsburgh, Pennsylvania	Minimum	69
	Maximum	385
	Average	180
Louisville, Kentucky	Minimum	74
	Maximum	415
	Average	176
Denver, Colorado	Minimum	36
	Maximum	471
	Average	131

It is estimated that the United States alone spews forth 200 million tons of aerial garbage each year.

In Paris, the residents' lungs have changed color. They are no longer the pinkish color they used to be. Instead, medical experts have noted while performing autopsies, the surface has a sort of blackish coating. This is one sign among so many others of the polluted Parisian air.

Astronomers at the Paris Observatory have given up using their telescopes to examine the sky because the air's transparency over the city has decreased by half. They now have to go to another observatory about six miles away.

In New York, the high levels of sulfur dioxide, produced by burning fuels, forced officials of the Metropolitan Museum of Art to coat priceless statuary with beeswax to prevent further deterioration.

Dr. E. Duhot made a survey of the toxic gases that hover over urban centers and are inhaled by city dwellers. The list is long. Nitric acid, nitrous acid, sulfuric acid, ammonia, hydrogen sulfide, and sulfur dioxide are present along with carbon monoxide, which has increased considerably over the past twenty years as a result of exhaust fumes from automobiles and smoke from factories.[3]

About one hundred tons of smoke fall every year on Paris. This smoke is produced by combustion from both domestic and industrial fires. Carbon, cinders, soot, tar, and water vapor are liberated from it, and these pollutants extend upward several hundred yards. According to J. Kohn-Abrest, a French toxicologist, "There is an actual canopy of smoke about one hundred yards above the earth, and the air there is even more polluted."

Dust particles, those mineral or vegetable particles that are the waste products of craft and industry, must also be included in the list of pollutants. They contain silica, ferric oxide, barium oxide, arsenious oxide, and pollen. It has been calculated that there are more than 100,000 grains of dust per cubic centimeter in the air of Paris as compared to only 500 per cubic centimeter over the Pacific Ocean.

The city dweller inhales a veritable culture of germs, especially molds and bacilli. Duhot points out that in a village near the Swiss border only one to four germs were counted per cubic centimeter. But in the heart of Paris there are 500 by 8 A.M. and 30,000 by 10 A.M. In the large Parisian department stores there are 50,000 germs per cubic centimeter, and this figure can reach 4 million when the stores are crowded before holidays!

For many years the municipal laboratory of Paris has been carefully examining the results of studies on atmospheric pollution. The standard tests concern the sulfuric acid and carbon monoxide levels in the air as well as the number of grains of dust. Two French physicians, Champollion and Raymond, have written on the very close connection between the annual curve representing the pollution of the Parisian air and the mortality rate.

3. E. Duhòt, *Les Climats et l'Organisme humain* (P.U.F.), p. 13.

Lung Cancer

The disasters at Liège, Donora, and London are accidents caused by exceptional meteorological conditions. These disasters cause alarm because of the high number of victims in a short period of time, victims who are primarily the ill, the elderly, and those with weak respiratory systems. But as Dr. P. J. Meade remarked, there exists a chronic state of atmospheric pollution. Its consequences are insidious and long-term, and therefore more dangerous than exceptional meteorological conditions. Atmospheric pollution carries with it the origins of deadly diseases that sometimes take years to develop and that can strike a man down in the prime of life. Lung cancer is unfortunately the best illustration of this.

Lung cancer is on the increase. At the present time in France it is responsible for more than ten thousand deaths per year, which is three times more than ten years ago. According to the American Cancer Society, lung cancer claimed 54,407 victims (45,383 men and 9,024 women) in the United States in 1967. It is estimated that 64,000 (53,100 men and 11,200 women) will die of this disease in 1971. Lung cancer deaths due to cigarette smoking are increasing steadily, especially among men, that death rate being now 15 times greater than it was 40 years ago. However, while there have been habitual smokers for a long time, the number of deaths from lung cancer has been increasing at an alarming rate only over the past ten years or so, and this increase can be seen proportionally among those persons who have never smoked. So excessive tobacco usage alone cannot adequately explain the upward spiral of this terrible disease.

The factors that aroused suspicion are the sprawling growth of urban areas and the increased atmospheric pollution from industrial expansion, which surrounds these areas with a belt of poisonous air. Recent studies by biometeorologists such as S. W. Tromp, Stocks, and S. Kreyberg suggest that the air we breathe is one of the most important etiological factors in the increased incidence of lung cancer. Numerous facts support this theory.

Murderous Cities

The number of deaths from lung cancer is considerably higher in cities and industrial areas than in rural areas. In the largest metropolitan areas of the United States, the death rate is twice that of rural sections. Significantly, the rate is generally in direct proportion to city population size as is, in general, the degree of air pollution. Even when lung cancer death rates are adjusted to take smoking habits and age into consideration, they are still a third higher in large cities than in rural areas.

A detailed study made in England also showed that the probability of a man dying from cancer of the lung increases in proportion to the number of inhabitants of the urban center where he lives. Between 1950 and 1953 the mortality rate for cancer of the lung was 64 deaths per 100,000 persons in rural districts. This figure increased to 84 in urban areas under 50,000 inhabitants; 93 in urban areas with 50,000–100,000 inhabitants; and 112 in urban areas with over 100,-000 inhabitants. A similar progression was noted by Tromp in the Netherlands, and by Kreyberg in Norway. These figures hold true for both the male and female populations.[4]

Studies by Stocks and Campbell show that the highest mortality from lung cancer does not occur in the cities where the most tobacco is consumed, but in those where the population density is the greatest. This is because heavily populated areas have a very high pollution index. Stocks draws

4. S. W. Tromp, "Cancer of the Lung," *Medical Biometeorology* (1963), p. 479.

another interesting observation from his data. It is not only the lungs that are irritated by the air's toxicity; the entire respiratory system is affected. In addition to lung cancer, frequent cases of cancer of the throat and trachea have been observed. Even the digestive tract suffers the consequences of pollution, although to a lesser degree; cancer of the esophagus and stomach is not rare in cities. On the other hand, population density does not affect the rate of cancer for those parts of the body that have had no contact with the contaminated air. Thus Stocks finds that city life has no bearing on the frequency of cancer of the breast or uterus in women.

Carcinogenic Substances in the Air

A large number of unrelated factors have been grouped together under the term "atmospheric pollution." Which of these factors should be considered the worst offender in pulmonary cancer?

The experts blame smoke, or more precisely, certain carbon compounds contained in the smoke, and they have furnished considerable proof of it. In the Netherlands Tromp noticed a distinct tendency for cancer to strike coal miners. A high incidence of scrotal cancer has been observed in chimney sweeps, who are constantly in contact with the by-products from the combustion of coal (tar, for example). Skin cancer occurs frequently among gas workers. Furthermore, the carcinogenic effect of tar has been proven in laboratory tests. Skin cancer, for example, has been induced by painting the skin of animals with extracts of coal tar.

These carcinogenic substances are present in the air of large cities. In 1930 Sir Ernest Kennaway and his co-workers succeeded in isolating one such substance, 3,4-benzpyrene. They showed that this product may be produced by pyrolysis (*i.e.* decomposition of organic substances in the air at high temperatures in the absence of oxygen). Extracts from air samples in Paris produce lung cancer in rats. These laboratory experiments are very disquieting because other equally harmful carcinogenic substances have been found in city air—namely 1,2-benzanthracene, 1,12-benzperylene, benzene, and arsenic.

There is now no doubt that it is not enough to abolish cigarette smoking to overcome lung cancer. It is also necessary to stop breathing contaminated city air. This is the heart of the problem.

Valuable Assistance from Meteorologists

There is essentially only one solution: reducing air pollution. But this will be a long struggle.

Many U.S. cities have air pollution alerts. In New York, for example, when the weather bureau advises that a high-pollution potential will exist for the next 24-48 hours, officials may shut down public and private incinerators, close garbage disposal plants and factories, and even ban automobiles if the situation warrants it. Los Angeles authorities are empowered to ban backyard barbecues when necessary.

E. W. Hewson has described how some experts in the United States and Canada have been able to control the daily emissions of toxic products from industrial plants in accordance with predicted meteorological conditions.[5] In the state of Washington manufacturers must drastically reduce the burning of waste products when there is very little wind and when dangerous fogs are likely to form over urban areas. The results have been excellent. Similar measures should be taken in all other densely populated areas.

5. E. W. Hewson, "Meteorological Control of Atmospheric Pollution by Heavy Industry," *Quart. J. Meteorol. Soc.*, 71 (1945), p. 266–82, 309.

Abolishing Pollution

It would be preferable to reduce the sources of pollution. Many cities now have ordinances requiring building owners to install anti-smoke filters on chimneys from central heating systems. In New York incinerators must be upgraded or discontinued; failure to comply results in fines or even jail sentences. Improper operation of incinerators and oil burners increase pollution, and New York now requires all persons who operate such equipment to be certified by the city's Department of Air Resources.

Sulphur emissions have been reduced 50 per cent in many cities by requiring the use of low sulphur content coal and fuel oil.

Cities faced with severe air pollution problems have taken steps to detect dangerous pollution levels. New York, for example, has a 38-station air monitoring network to provide a continuous profile of the air quality in virtually every neighborhood in the city, and it is only one of many cities which have a special telephone number for citizens to report excessive smoke and incinerator emissions.

More than half of Los Angeles' air pollution problem is caused by automotive exhaust. To combat this, exhaust controls have been mandatory there on all new vehicles beginning with the 1966 models. In 1970, the United States Congress passed legislation requiring emission control devices on cars beginning with 1978 models, and *by 1976 all new cars must have low emission engines* (i.e., a 90 per cent reduction of hydrocarbons, carbon monoxide, and nitrogen oxides).

Architects are becoming increasingly aware of the importance of meteorological problems for the health of city dwellers. "Urban planning bureaus" have been created to deal with these problems. They emphasize the numerous benefits of parks and green open spaces, which reduce the pollution level, diminish germs and dust, increase the amount of oxygen in the air, and decrease the carbon dioxide level. Urban specialists foresee many more parks in the cities of tomorrow.

In the future, various parts of a city must be laid out "functionally." Urban planners will have to bear in mind the direction of the prevailing winds when considering the distribution of industrial and residential zones. In Paris, where the prevailing wind is westerly, it would obviously be advisable for all the factories to be located east of the city. Thus the smoke and waste products would be dispersed over rural areas instead of over the city.

Urban planners are also considering separate traffic routes for automobiles and pedestrians. It is very important to reduce the constant inhalation of gasoline exhaust fumes by pedestrians. Automobile-free shopping malls are desirable for health as well as esthetic reasons.

To prevent the recurrence of tragedies like those at Liège, Donora, and London and to stop the increasing incidence of cancer of the respiratory system, the cooperation of specialists and the efforts of government and private citizens are both desirable and necessary.

Compass Card

"He who knows the origin of the winds, of thunder, and of the weather also knows where diseases come from," stated the great doctor Paracelsus at the beginning of the sixteenth century. All of us feel the effects of wind on our bodies. When the wind blows we become anxious and ill at ease. So, while a lack of wind is dangerous over cities, strong winds can be just as harmful. The dry, icy northeast wind grips us, and the heavy, humid wind coming from the tropics is oppressive.

One wind is universally more dangerous than all others:

this is the very warm, dry wind. It manifests itself in countless ways and bears many names according to each locale. In the south of Italy it is known as *sirocco*, "father of depression." In Spain it is called *leveccio*. It is the *chamsin* in Egypt, the *simoun* in the Sahara, the *zonda* in Argentina, and the *chinook* in the United States. But there are two winds, the Austrian *foehn* and the *autan* of France, whose effects on man have been extensively studied by doctors.

The Snow Swallower

The word *foehn* dates back to the Middle Ages. This wind was called the *phoenicias* in the gilded manuscripts of the Renaissance because men believed that it came from Phoenicia.[6] The name was subsequently abbreviated to *foehn*. It is a southerly wind which comes from Italy, carrying masses of humid air toward the Swiss Alps. The impact cools it, and heavy precipitation results. The air mass, still warm but dried out, then descends into the northern valleys of the Alps. The mountain people dread the foehn because it causes avalanches in winter. It has been called "the snow swallower," because its warmth causes snow to melt or sometimes even evaporate without forming a stream.

After passing the Alps, the foehn heads toward Innsbruck in Austria. Its arrival is accompanied by a large drop in barometric pressure which often extends beyond Innsbruck and encompasses the entire Tyrol and all of Austria and Switzerland.

As soon as the foehn starts blowing, and sometimes even as it is approaching, people exhibit the typical symptoms of irritability, headaches, anxiety, insomnia, and nightmares. Its approach is a bad omen for the sick. Countless German,

6. B. de Rudder, *Grundriss einer Meteorobiologie des Menschen* (1952), p. 26.

Austrian, and Swiss doctors have described the breathing difficulties of cardiac patients and the restlessness of nervous persons. The crime rate and the number of suicides increase. The detrimental effects of the foehn are felt to such an extent in Central Europe that warning of its arrival creates a type of panic called "foehn psychosis." Even before it starts to blow, some people experience reactions to it, but these are products of the imagination. Nevertheless, the foehn's reputation cannot be denied.

The Autan

This wind blows up the Rhone valley in eastern France. It is a strong, warm wind accompanied by a temperature increase and by a decrease in humidity and pressure, which has intense effects. In some ways, it is a twin brother to the foehn. Prof. Georges Mouriquand of Lyon has very accurately described these peculiar biological effects.[7]

He noticed that infants are the first to show symptoms of distress when the autan blows. In mild cases the baby is simply restless, anxious, and unable to sleep. In nurseries the infants' cries sometimes become piercing and stop only when the wind changes direction.

If these symptoms become worse, we then see the real "south wind syndrome" described by Mouriquand: "There is a considerable rise in temperature accompanied by dehydration and serious nutritional disorders. This situation quickly becomes serious, . . . resembling, in short, neurotoxic cases." He adds: "Luckily this type of reaction is rare. It is observed mainly in young children who are already sensitized because of inadequate nutrition or because of previous illnesses, such as toxic infections. It can even result in death

7. George Mouriquand, "Remarques sur les météopathies," *Maroc Médical,* no. 342 (November 1953).

in extreme cases. But if the wind stops or else 'turns to the north,' then veritable resurrections are apparent."

The symptoms become less marked as the child gets older. But they can persist in children who are predisposed to them. Their reactions take various forms. The least affected simply become irritable and usually get poor school reports because of restlessness and inattention in class. According to Mouriquand, "There is a rain of punishment in school when the autan blows at Lyon." Some children break out in hives. Others suffer respiratory ailments, simple colds, and occasionally asthma attacks. Digestive complaints have also been observed, such as a coated tongue, stomachaches, and vomiting. Once again, these symptoms disappear rapidly as soon as the wind abates.

In adults the "south wind" is notorious for causing weakness and irritability. People start quarreling at home and in the streets. Insomnia is a frequent symptom. Cardiac patients, and coronary patients in particular, are susceptible to its effects. Those who are afflicted with migraine, rheumatism, and neuralgia also suffer. Professor M. Piéry noted an increased frequency of spitting up blood in patients with tuberculosis. Professor Poncet, a surgeon, has noticed that the condition of patients who have undergone surgery suddenly becomes critical. When the autan blows, they often develop unexpected complications.

An interesting phenomenon is that the morbid manifestations occasionally precede the wind's arrival. Some people are "south wind" prophets. Professor Mouriquand mentions the case of one of his patients with a liver disease who used to vomit bile when the autan was still a half-mile high and detectable only by sounding balloons. We shall understand the reason for this reaction soon.

The Mistral and the Tramontana

Northerly winds have never been the object of such detailed studies. Yet they also have serious effects on our health.

The mistral is a violent northerly wind of southeastern France, especially prevalent along the Rhône valley. Not only does it cause migraine and insomnia, but it can also provoke a sudden recurrence of previous neuralgia. It is often accompanied by cold spells that are particularly hazardous for pulmonary patients. Dr. Daremburg observed that the mistral causes tubercular patients to be congested and cough blood.

The tramontana, another northerly Mediterranean wind, produces similar effects.

How can we explain this disturbing role of the wind on the human organism? In reality, it is not the blowing of the wind that affects us because the walls of houses provide adequate shelter, but the sudden meteorological variations accompanying the wind. The changes of temperature, pressure, humidity, and electrical potential cause the clinical symptoms mentioned above by upsetting the body's hormone balance and the vascular system. We shall have a better understanding of these phenomena when we have studied how meteorological fronts pass, a study fundamental to an understanding of biometeorology.

Weather Prophets

All of us have heard or have said ourselves at one time: "The weather is going to change soon. I can feel it in my bones." There are a thousand possible variations of this saying, but the assertion remains the same: namely, that the weather is going to change. It seems that some sensitive people actually have the mysterious ability to predict weather changes one or two days before they occur. In France these people are called "weather prophets." In Germany doctors have termed them *"Wettervogel"* or "weatherbirds."

It is interesting to note that this is one of the oldest medical observations. Hippocratic medicine mentions pains preceding changes of weather. In the Middle Ages they were mentioned in judicial decrees. In the *Lex Frisionum,* the civil and penal code of Western Friesland in the ninth century, we can read: "Inflicting a wound will be punished with a stronger fine if it leaves a scar which is sensitive to changes of weather." Several fourteenth-century manuscripts mention, in chapters on taxes and fines, that the sentence is heavier if the plaintiff's wounds cause him pain when the weather is changing. A significant police report dates from the sixteenth century. A student at the University of Ingolstadt in Bavaria was treated so roughly by nightwatchmen "that he bears several wounds on his head. Now, when the weather is about to change, he experiences such pains that he is unable to study." The court awarded him a substantial sum as compensation.

This "advance knowledge" of a change in the weather varies from one individual to another. There are some exceptionally gifted weather prophets. Dr. J. Bauer of Frankfurt mentions the case of a female patient whom he followed every day for many years. "She never made a mistake in predicting what the weather was going to be," he asserts.

Dr. de Rudder loves to relate the story of one of his colleagues who had a scar at the apex of the lung and who maintained that this scar could inform him of future weather changes. De Rudder was skeptical. One winter day the two men were walking together along a street in Frankfurt. The sky was perfectly clear and blue.

"I can feel that it's going to snow tomorrow," said his colleague.

The weather was so beautiful that this did not seem likely

to de Rudder. But eighteen hours later the snow began to fall. There was a bad storm with heavy snow and fierce winds.[8] De Rudder's colleague was an extraordinary "weatherbird." But not everyone is so gifted.

A healthy, robust, and well-balanced person is rarely sensitive to changes of weather. Weather-sensitive individuals seem to have special temperaments. Generally speaking, they suffer from chronic diseases that react painfully to barometric variations. Drs. L. Miller and A. Farkas wrote: "Patients who have chronic pain in their joints, patients with tabes, hemiplegia, and those with scars or stumps from amputated limbs react to changes of weather. They complain of *drawing* and *tearing* sensations a short time before the bad weather arrives, usually two days before." [9] Rheumatism sufferers are the most affected. They experience pain with the slightest weather change. But persons who have had fractures, dislocations, and burns are also affected. After the wounds have healed, pain recurs whenever the weather is about to change. This pain attenuates over the years but never completely disappears. Chafed areas or even common corns can also act as barometers.

One German doctor reported a strange case. One of his patients had lost a leg during World War I. Whenever the weather was changing, he felt pain, not in the stump, but in a corn he had had on one of his toes before the leg was amputated.

All these empirical observations conceal a real medical mystery. What happens in the systems of weather-sensitive persons? What strange meteorological phenomena are buried in the vague expression "change of weather"? Biometeorologists have done much more than lift a corner of the mysterious curtain. But if we are to understand their discoveries, we must first make a short excursion into meteorology.

8. De Rudder, *op. cit.*, p. 46.
9. *Ibid.*, p. 45.

Air Masses

The classical methods of measuring temperature, humidity, wind velocity, and atmospheric pressure no longer suffice. The modern meteorologist is concerned with more global concepts. The very important idea of "air mass" was formulated by a school of Norwegian meteorologists, Bjerknes, Solberg, and Bergeron, and it encompasses all the classical methods of measurement.

An air mass is a large quantity of air with roughly the same physical and chemical properties, extending over hundreds or even thousands of miles and reaching a depth of more than one-half mile. An air mass never originates over temperate zones, where there is constant atmospheric turbulence, but at the poles or at the equator when conditions there are calm.

The air mass remains at its place of origin acquiring the climatic properties typical of that region. Then, for obscure reasons, it starts to move. It becomes a sort of "moving climate," imposing its climatic characteristics on the areas over which it passes. It differs in every respect from the surrounding air it meets, which it gradually replaces.

New air masses, brought by various winds, reach us regularly, making our weather quite unstable. The north wind brings masses of polar air that is cold and humid when it comes from Greenland but cold and dry when it comes from Siberia. The south wind brings masses of tropical air that is warm and dry when it comes from Africa but temperate and moist when it comes from the Azores.

When two air masses meet, the mass that was prevailing is pushed away or "kicked out" by the incoming mass. They do not mix. The warm air, which has a tendency to rise, more or less covers the cold air. But they are not superimposed like oil and water; there is a dividing line between the two air masses that forms an acute angle with the ground. Meteorologists call this dividing line a "front." As one air mass displaces another, we say that "a front is passing." What modern meteorologists call a "passing front" corresponds to the "change in the weather" formerly used by weather forecasters. If warm air moves toward an area with cold air, we say a "warm front" is approaching; conversely, if cold air moves toward a warm area, it is called a "cold front."

Dramatic Upheavals

It is the incompatibility of two air masses of opposite character that makes the phenomenon of a passing front so dramatic and brutal. From one day to the next, with almost no transition, we can pass from cold weather to warm weather or vice versa. The contrast in temperature is often greater than 25° F. This causes other meteorological factors to be disturbed proportionally. The front is accompanied by severe atmospheric turbulence, affecting the wind, barometric pressure, humidity, and many other factors that have not yet been defined.

These disturbances have a marked influence on our bodies. They would not be so severe if the air masses mixed, but they do not. From one day to the next, without even leaving our homes, we literally change climates. Anyone who has experienced, on leaving a plane, the shock of encountering a new climate without any transition can readily comprehend that the passing of fronts is linked to the appearance of numerous symptoms.

The meteorological war between two air masses, each trying to displace the other, lasts about twenty-four hours before the invading air mass wins. This fact explains the abilities of "weather prophets." Their hypersensitive systems are capable of perceiving before anyone else the first advance signs of the battle.

A healthy person does not react as quickly or as precisely to the passing of a front as a "weather prophet." Nevertheless, most of the physiological processes in the human body are constantly being modified by climate and weather. The characteristics of the blood change. Blood clotting occurs faster just before a front passes. Fibrinolysis, or the dissolution of blood clots, definitely increases with the passage of cold fronts. Diuresis, or the amount of urine produced, increases while cold fronts are passing, but decreases after a tropical air mass has passed. The endocrine glands are also affected. The blood-sugar level is altered, as are the levels of calcium, phosphates, sodium, and magnesium. "It is easy to imagine all the possible consequences of these phenomena in some diseases," concludes Rivolier.

What is interesting is that these phenomena generally occur during the passing of both warm and cold fronts. In effect, the body's regulatory systems are overcome by atmospheric disturbances caused when fronts are passing. These fronts act aggressively on the body, often producing serious effects. This is what Hans Seylie, an American biologist, has termed "the state of stress." If a healthy person is so strongly affected by weather changes, it is easy to understand how the consequences of a state of stress can become dangerous for a sick person.

Episodes of Illness

General practitioners in their daily rounds sometimes see serious "episodes of illness" with no apparent external cause. These do not include epidemics caused by infectious agents, but are a series of emergencies with no direct links to each other. A doctor can be called ten times in forty-eight hours to patients suddenly suffering myocardial infarction, or patients with angina pectoris who are having choking spells. During the same period he may be called for a severe gallstone attack and a cerebral hemorrhage. Then, after this dramatic accumulation of illness, everything calms down until the next "episode."

What causes these "episodes"? They generally occur during sudden changes of weather. The passing of a front is the most disturbing meteorological factor where health is concerned. Even benign maladies recur at this time. In January 1966, after a very cold week, a tropical air mass suddenly approached and warmed the Parisian atmosphere. At that moment a violent epidemic broke out, coupled with a particularly painful type of angina. It is commonly acknowledged that colds and influenza strike more severely during sudden warm spells in winter. On the other hand, when a polar air mass suddenly lowers the thermometer several degrees, pneumonia becomes a threat.

There are countless incidents of these episodic outbreaks of illness. Statistical studies confirm current medical observations. Doctor Hüttl Tivadar from Budapest established that cardiac attacks are twice as common on days when fronts are passing. In Pomerania, Drs. H. Raettig and H. Nehls found similar results by studying the dates on which 489 cardiac emboli occurred. In these cases cold fronts are the deadliest. A urologist from Leipzig, Dr. Ernst Hauck, recorded the days when his patients suffered acute occlusion of the renal and urinary ducts by stones or hypertrophy of the prostate. These ailments occurred "in groups" on days when the weather changed. He counted 316 cases on the day a front was passing, but only 189 the day before and 195 the day after.

Surgical Complications

Surgeons know that complications occur more frequently at certain times. There is always the risk of complications during an operation, but the greatest dangers are post-operative accidents such as sudden hemorrhage and cardiac embolization. All these accidents are linked to alterations in the blood-clotting mechanism. Anesthetists, who have great responsibility during the operation itself, are always on the alert for these. One anesthetist reports that there are some days when it is very difficult to anesthetize patients, and when patients stay in a disturbed state of post-anesthetic restlessness.

Extensive medical studies concerning this problem have been conducted in several European countries. The most interesting were performed in Germany. Dr. J. Kümmel's 1936 study is a classic one. He concludes that operations are the most dangerous when the weather is changing.[10] Another investigator, Dr. E. Rappert, undertook an imposing experiment. In "Post-Operative Complications and the Weather" he reports that he studied 2,100 surgical cases in Vienna over a period of a year.[11] Of these 2,100 cases, 386 had complications, all of which occurred in groups.

90 percent of the "groups" occurred during a change in the weather

10 percent occurred during stable weather

60 percent coincided with the approach of a cold front

30 percent coincided with the approach of a warm front

10. J. Kümmel, "Operationsgefährdung," *Zbl. Chirurgie* (1936), p. 1023.

11. E. Rappert, "Postoperative Komplikationen und Wetter," *Deut. Zschrift für Chirurgie,* no. 244, p. 537.

Rappert concluded his report by advising surgeons to consider the weather and to consult weather bureaus in order to be aware of coming conditions. In this way, they could decide the best time for surgery that is not urgent.

Surgery should be avoided, if possible, when the weather is changing. If an emergency does arise when there is considerable atmospheric turbulence, more stringent precautionary measures should be taken to avoid subsequent complications. Thus, collaboration between meteorologists and surgeons is highly recommended.

Rheumatism and Weather Changes

Rheumatism is a very widespread affliction in temperate countries. Thirty percent of the illness in Sweden and the Netherlands is due to one form or another of rheumatism, especially in the fifty-and-older age group. In 1966 about 11 million people in the United States were suffering from this disease. Of these, 300,000 were temporarily unemployable. In Great Britain 440 million pounds sterling are lost every year due to rheumatic illness. In France the figures are just as pessimistic. In spite of cortisone treatment, millions of Frenchmen are still afflicted with rheumatism.

It is true that rheumatic diseases are not a sharply defined group; so many varied ailments are classified as rheumatism. "Medically speaking," writes Rivolier, "there can be no comparison between chronic (migrating) polyarthritis and an attack of acute articular rheumatism." The classical symptoms of rheumatism are usually described as a condition affecting the connective tissues, marked by stiffness in joints, muscles, and related structures. The pain associated with this disease is generally intermittent.

Here is where weather changes play their most significant role. It would take an entire book to mention all the research that has been done on the effects of weather on rheumatism. An infinite number of medical theories exist, of which the following are very typical.

In 1931 Drs. W. Feige and R. Freund utilized the vast quantity of statistical material gathered by the Breslauer Krankenkasse (Breslau Health Insurance Bureau). Thanks to this early form of social security, they were able to establish that rheumatic attacks severe enough to cause a subject to stop work were definitely related to the passing of fronts. Tromp conducted a more recent and complete study. From November 1956 to July 1958 he followed a group of thirty-five out-patient rheumatics on a daily basis and concluded: "The most harmful meteorological events are a sudden drop in temperature, strong winds, and the influx of polar air masses.[12] Dr. H. Ungleheuer likewise observed that the sharper the weather change, the more severe the complaints.

What happens to a patient when the weather changes? Dr. Kurt Franke found important structural modifications in the skin capillaries of rheumatics during changes of weather. Similar observations were made by Dr. Bettmann who noticed vaso-motor changes in the skin capillaries of patients. These changes disappear and the capillary pattern becomes normal again when the weather stabilizes. Observations like these have doubtless contributed to the development of climatic treatments for rheumatic diseases. These treatments have proven a very useful substitute in some cases for certain medications.

Acute Asthma Attacks

An incident that took place on the night of August 8–August 9, 1931, and extended all over Europe was reported by two Dutch doctors, Storm van Leeuwen and Wijn-

12. S. W. Tromp: "Rheumatic Diseases" (*op. cit.* p. 549).

gaarden.[13] On that night numerous people suddenly acquired a severe but non-infectious cold. Some of them had not had colds for years; furthermore, it was summer, an unusual time for colds. Of the 4,528 persons subsequently interrogated, 11 percent had been affected.

On that same night most asthma sufferers in France, Germany, Belgium, and the Netherlands suffered serious attacks. Even passengers on boats crossing the English Channel that night were affected. Yet the most acute asthmatics experienced nothing *if* they happened to be in air-conditioned hospital rooms.

No one has been able to determine exactly what happened that night. Doctors regret that it is now impossible to know what meteorological conditions prevailed in Europe at the time. But they assume that a front, extending from England to Italy, moved in very rapidly. They feel certain that the weather was the cause of the asthma attacks.

The characteristics of a bronchial asthma attack are as follows. It usually begins with a general feeling of breathlessness. Then sibilant and sonorous rales are heard throughout the afflicted patient's chest. He struggles to catch his breath and does so with great difficulty. The attack may be intermittent or continuous with exacerbations of varying degree. The breathing difficulty is the result of a long, physiologically abnormal process. The bronchi and bronchioles are obstructed by an exaggerated contraction of the smooth muscle fibers of the bronchi. This contraction is initiated by an abnormal stimulation of the parasympathetic nervous system, or by excessive production of contractile substances like histamine.

Asthma is a very widespread ailment, with a high incidence among children. In the United States, approximately 6 million people suffer from asthma, of whom half are chil-

13. Storm van Leeuwen and Wijngaarden, "Asthma, Bronchitis und Schnupfen in Zusammenhang mit der Jahreszeit," *Münch. Med. Wschr.* (1932), p. 583.

dren under 17. Studies in European countries indicate that 6 per 1000 children suffer from it. For the adult population, the figure is even greater: 9 adults per 1000 in Holland, and 14 per 1000 in Sweden. We are already familiar with several allergic or psychological causes of asthma and the influence of the weather, only recently discovered, must also be added to the list.

A Great Offender—the Weather

What factors most often cause asthma attacks? Tromp answered this question after conducting a ten-year study on asthmatic children and adults. Whenever one of his patients had an attack, he recorded all the environmental conditions prevailing at that time. When after ten years he analyzed the voluminous data he had compiled, he found that the most frequent link with asthma attacks was the passing of weather fronts. Cold fronts, in particular, always provoke an outbreak of asthma attacks. Fog, on the other hand, has no asthma-producing effect, contrary to what was previously believed. Allergies due to pollen in the air exist, but their connection with asthma attacks is less clear than it used to be. However, Tromp did observe that asthma frequency follows a seasonal rhythm that is high in summer and autumn, but low in winter. The longest and most distressing attacks occur in June.

As with so many other diseases, atmospheric turbulence resulting from a change in weather appears primarily responsible for asthma attacks. Thus, when the weather is going to change, patients should pay particular attention and keep medication available in order to prevent or alleviate a possible attack.*

* See the Appendix.

Acute Glaucoma Attacks

The influence of weather changes can be seen in other diseases that are rarer than asthma and rheumatism—for example, acute glaucoma.

Glaucoma is a serious eye disease, characterized by excessive intraocular pressure which causes severe pain radiating from the eye to the upper jaws and head. If it is not treated in time, glaucoma can cause partial or total loss of vision in the affected eye.

In 1930 Dr. Loeffler published a report on the occurrence of glaucoma attacks. She wrote: "I have compiled abundant clinical material in Vienna and have discovered distinct periods when acute glaucoma attacks occur. The highest incidence coincides with the passage of weather fronts, particularly during sudden warming trends in winter and sudden drops of temperature in summer." [14]

Dr. H. Fischer's recent study shows that glaucoma attacks are three times more frequent on days when fronts are passing than on calm days. All doctors who have studied this problem confirm the relationship between weather and acute glaucoma.

Protecting our Lives

The biometeorologist de Rudder states: "Mortality often increases while fronts are passing." In the opinion of many biometeorologists, the passage of fronts is the most alarming meteorological influence on our health. However, there is nothing new about this fact. The weather's effect on our

14. De Rudder, *op. cit.*, p. 61.

health has always existed, but now our knowledge of this phenomenon is becoming greater.

Today, for example, we know that a "cold spell" means much more than a mere drop in temperature. It is always accompanied by complex modifications of barometric pressure, wind direction, and humidity. All these changes affect our bodies, upset our endocrine systems, and influence our blood vessels and nervous systems.

People in good health experience only a passing feeling of discomfort. But for the sick person whose system is weakened, for someone who has undergone major surgery, or for those with high blood pressure, the feeling of discomfort can become something much more critical.

By knowing the effects of the environmental atmosphere on the human organism, doctors are able to warn us of potential danger. The studies by meteorologists of air masses and approaching fronts have greatly advanced medical knowledge and so aid in the protection of our lives.

The Consequences of Storms

The summer day had been not only hot, but also oppressive. The evening was stifling. Heavy gray clouds covered the sky over the parched countryside. Farm animals were restless. Not a sound could be heard, and there was not a breath of wind. Insects were flying unusually low, and birds were skimming the ground as they pursued them. A storm was approaching. City dwellers were tense and ill at ease. Some were finding it difficult to breathe, some were perspiring, and others had developed migraine.

At last the wind rose, the thunder growled, and lightning went zigzagging across the sky. Then the welcome rain began to fall, bringing relief to both man and animal.

Storms are one of the most spectacular meteorological

phenomena. For many years doctors have recognized count-less morbid pre-storm symptoms. For example, patients with angina pectoris experience difficulty, there is a recurrence of emboli and spitting up blood in tubercular patients, and asthmatics suffer attacks of breathlessness.

Pre-storm symptoms in infants, as described by A. Lesage, are restlessness, insomnia, and incessant crying. De Rudder found a correlation between the number of storms and the ravages of the diphtheria epidemic in Germany during the summer of 1926.

The role of electricity in the atmosphere is primarily re-sponsible for starting storms and for provoking the morbid symptoms accompanying them. As the storm clouds approach, there is an abnormal variation in the potential gradient of the atmosphere, which in turn modifies the balance of bodily functions.

Lightning, which still kills or injures thousands of people every year, is the visible and brutal manifestation of the abnormal electrical state in the atmosphere before and dur-ing storms. But the effect of lightning is a mechanical one: with an electrical discharge with an intensity of 100,000 amperes and a tension of millions of volts, it electrocutes any victim found in its path; its action, however, is limited and accidental.

Variations of the potential gradient produced in storms can influence the body in much more subtle ways. Some specialists have experienced these effects personally. Arsène d'Arsonval, a French biologist, made the following observa-tion: "I always feel oppressed just before a storm. But this malaise disappears if I sit on an insulated stool with a field established between myself and the negative pole of an acti-vated electrostatic machine. On the other hand, my discom-fort increases if I establish a field between myself and the positive pole."

Another interesting account is that of a doctor from Besançon. One stormy day he suffered cardiac palpitations.

Then he noticed a strange coincidence, namely that his palpitations synchronized perfectly with electrical discharges from the atmosphere which he detected as interference on his radio set.

Electricity in the Air

When a storm is approaching, people often say, "There is a lot of electricity in the air." But this expression is incorrect. There is always electricity in the air; without it we could not live. This vital discovery, made only recently, has enabled us to see the importance of electron exchanges in phenomena associated with life. We were already familiar with molecular exchanges, which permit the chemical resources of our bodies to function. But more complex still are electron exchanges, which form a network of subtle electrical connections.

For example, we have observed that infants kept in electrically isolated cribs gain more weight than those in unisolated cribs. Rivolier states that although the mechanism involved is still not fully understood, "When considering biometeorological elements, atmospheric electricity undeniably attracts our attention. We are tempted to see the quality and quantity of electrical charges in the air as a direct cause of physiopathological changes." [15]

Dr. André Dussert from Bergerac cites a really dramatic experience along these lines. One of his colleagues, aged fifty-five, suffered from high blood pressure. After a very busy week of work, he had to make a business trip. After spending the whole night on a train, he took a car at 4 A.M. and traveled about 200 miles. At 10 A.M. he started climbing with a rucksack on his back toward Lake Gaube in the Pyrenees. After walking for an hour, he fell down dead.

15. Rivolier, *op. cit.*, p. 26.

At that very moment, Dr. Dussert's meteorological instruments detected an electrically positive storm with a potential gradient of 800 to 1,000 volts per meter approaching the entire Pyrenees region.

The atmosphere is constantly in an electric field. This means that there is a difference of potential between any two points. The field is oriented vertically. In fine weather the earth has a positive charge, and the base of the clouds a negative charge. So the field is normally oriented from top to bottom. But during certain periods the current reverses itself. The average difference in potential is 100 volts per meter. In the dramatic case reported by Dussert, this potential suddenly increased tenfold. This is what caused the fatal accident to his exhausted colleague.

Large fluctuations of the electrical potential are directly linked to potential meteorological phenomena. They bring about rain, snow, and fog. Winds, too, play an extremely important role in this respect.

In 1960 Dr. J. C. Jardel published a very interesting thesis on the effect of variations of electrical potential on sick persons. Every day for two years Jardel observed patients who were receiving treatment in several French sanatoria. The majority of their relapses almost always coincided with major, prolonged fluctuations of electrical potential on earth. On these turbulent days Jardel recorded more cases of migraine, insomnia, various pains, asthma attacks, etc.

What happens in the human body when these fluctuations occur? Biologists think that our physiological exchanges are disturbed by the invasion of groups of electrified particles that are stronger than usual. It is important to note that the effect varies according to whether the particles are electrically positive or negative.

Harmful Ions and Beneficial Ions

The air we breathe contains electrified particles known as "ions." For a long time these ions were a mystery, but we are now beginning to understand them.

Ions are atoms or molecules that have gained or lost an electron. Negative ions are those that have gained an electron, and positive ions are those that have lost one. The number of positive and negative ions in the atmosphere varies according to season, time of day, atmospheric purity, and, especially, meteorological conditions. The atmosphere is therefore filled with these electrified particles, but the positive-negative balance is constantly changing. Sometimes positive ions predominate; at other times negative ions predominate. These electric charges have a considerable influence on biological exchanges.

Generally speaking, positive ions are detrimental to our health and well-being. When the air is full of positive ions, we experience discomforts. One of the first men to discover this was Prof. A. L. Tchjewsky of Moscow, who noted that positive ions can have a depressing effect. A comprehensive study made in the United States by T. Winsor and J. Beckett proved the harmfulness of positive ions. These researchers asked a number of volunteers to inhale air containing 32 million positive ions per cubic centimeter for 20 minutes. At the end of the experiment, every subject complained of dizziness and obstruction of the throat. Their nasal mucosa were irritated and dry, and their voices were hoarse.[16]

Dr. Dussert concluded that an excess of positive ions in the air we breathe is responsible for a large number of indispositions. In the USSR several studies have proven the unfavorable influence of an excess of positive air ions in

16. T. Winsor and J. Beckett, "Biological Effects of Ionized Air on Man," *Am. J. Physic. Med.*, no. 37 (1958), p. 83.

cardiac problems and surgical complications. Soviet doctors have been able to diminish the risk in the latter case by neutralizing the number of positive ions in operating rooms by using a machine that emits a scientifically regulated number of electrons.

On the other hand, an abundance of negative air ions is generally beneficial. Respiration becomes easier, biological exchanges are favorably stimulated, and the subject feels euphoric.

Doctors are very enthusiastic about the results obtained from experiments with animals. When exposed to high densities of negative ions, rats become more active and chickens grow faster. The results on man are just as surprising. I. H. Kornblueh, an American, has gained world renown in this field. He has treated more than two hundred victims of third-degree burns with negative air ions and has been able to stop their pain and prevent infection from developing in their wounds. He has improved the condition of persons suffering from hay fever by making them inhale negative ions. He feels that this treatment also diminishes the risks of post-operative complications. After analyzing brain waves on electroencephalograms, Kornblueh and his colleague Silvermann have concluded that negative air ions have a tranquilizing action on the brain.

Heavy Ions in Cities

The respiratory system is the organ most sensitive to atmospheric ions. A P. Krueger and R. F. Smith, two American doctors, believe that there is an association between the number of positive air ions inhaled and lung cancer. Inhalation of positive ions decreases the activity of the vibratory cilia of the bronchi. Their beating rate can drop from 850 to only 350 beats per minute, thus preventing the bronchi from completely dispelling the carcinogenic substances inhaled with tobacco smoke or with particles from the cities' polluted atmosphere. On the other hand, inhaling negative ions assists and increases vibratory ciliary activity. Krueger and Smith concluded: "Perhaps one day negative ion generators will become as popular as cigarette filters." [17] The Germans installed such generators in their submarines during World War II in order to facilitate the crew's respiration.

Controlling the ion density in the air we breathe seems extremely useful. Some meteorological factors such as wind or fog can influence the positive air ion concentration, causing it to become dangerously high over cities.

Unfortunately for city dwellers, cities generate enormous quantities of excess positive air ions. Exhaust fumes from cars, smoke, and dust cause these ions to cluster in large molecules. They are the "heavy ions," discovered by French physicist Paul Langevin, which hover over the earth's surface. They have rightly been named "killing ions." The catastrophes at Liège, Donora, and London mentioned previously were caused by these ions. They are likewise believed responsible for the air's toxicity. Indirectly they are probably responsible for the increase in lung cancer because they decrease the flow of tracheal mucosa, thus slowing down the elimination of carcinogenic substances.

A Panacea?

Once we know the evil, a remedy is possible. Air ions offer us a fresh chance to improve health conditions and protect ourselves from the evils of atmospheric pollution. Participants at a recent convention in Chicago reached this

17. A. P. Krueger and R. F. Smith, "An Enzymatic Basis for the Acceleration of Ciliary Activity of Negative Air Ions," *Nature*, no. 183, (1959), p. 1332.

conclusion: "It seems reasonable to predict that in the future we shall see the development of atmospheric ion control at home and at work, just as we now control temperature and humidity." [18]

There is already one research center at Nashville, Ohio, which is developing instruments capable of neutralizing the harmful ions by burning the carbon particles contained in the gasoline exhaust fumes of automobiles. It is hoped that these devices will be made compulsory in the United States as soon as they have been perfected.

In the USSR negative air-ion clinics have been created where people may go and inhale the salutary air, and in France some medical services are using ionization in the treatment of several diseases, especially rheumatic pain and muscular trauma.

But the inhalation of negative air ions should not be regarded as a universal panacea. In the Soviet Union, where this type of treatment is very popular, citizens have been warned against making their own negative air-ion generators. They are not easy machines to construct, and should only be used under medical supervision. The theoretical concept of the beneficial influence of ions still has to be studied in depth because individuals differ with regard to air-ion sensitivity. There have even been cases of patients relieved by the presence of positive air ions.

However, the concept does offer hope in the fight against the adverse effects of unhealthy meteorological conditions and their accomplice, atmospheric pollution.

Strange Long Waves

In 1953, at the Munich Traffic Exhibition, about 53,000 visitors participated in a reaction-time test, unaware that

18. A. P. Krueger and R. F. Smith, "Positive and Negative Ionization of the Atmosphere," *Man's Dependence on the Earthly Atmosphere*, p. 362.

some time later two researchers would analyze the results and make an important discovery. In one of the stands at the exhibition there was a machine measuring reaction time. The subject held a lever, and when a light suddenly flashed on, he had to turn it off as quickly as he could by lowering the lever. The time interval between the appearance of the light and the subject's reaction was recorded.

Two physicists, R. Reiter and H. Koenig, examined the recorded reaction times and noted some strange coincidences. There were some days when all the visitors reacted rapidly and other days when every subject was slow and clumsy. Reiter and Koenig tried to account for these differences and came up with this explanation. The "off" days were those when the atmosphere was disturbed by the presence of very long, low-frequency electromagnetic waves. Man is considerably influenced by these long waves. His manual dexterity changes. Drivers, for example, run a greater risk of having an accident on days when very high electromagnetic impulses are recorded.

The presence of long waves in the atmosphere is closely linked to the weather. These waves are emitted at the approach of low pressure areas and storms. They are more frequent in spring, diminish in winter, and almost always accompany tropical air masses.

How do these waves act on the human organism? Koenig and another colleague, F. Ankermüller, placed a group of test subjects in an air-tight room and subjected them to an artificial field of electromagnetic long waves. After spending a few moments in this environment, the subjects described what they felt. Some stated that they had bad headaches. Others felt perspiration forming on the palms of their hands. Others felt tired and complained of feeling weight on their chests.[19]

The electrical exchanges of our bodies are therefore in-

19. H. Koenig and F. Ankermüller, "Ueber den Einfluss besonders niederfrequenter elektrischer Vorgänge in der Atmosphäre auf dem Menschen," *Naturwissenschaften*, no. 21, (1960), p. 486.

fluenced by the presence of very long electromagnetic waves in the atmosphere. And since these electromagnetic impulses are related to the weather, this discovery could be very important in preventing accidents on the road and at work. When more precise meteorological data become available, we will be able to warn the public in advance of the probable arrival of these dreaded waves: "Beware! Tomorrow be doubly careful on the road and at work. Your reflexes will probably be slower and less well coordinated than usual."

Thus discovering the biological role of electromagnetic long waves adds another chapter to the strange effects of atmospheric electricity on our health.

Physical Constitution and the Weather

The following problem occurs regularly where several people work together in an office. When the central heating is on, one person is too hot and wants to open a window, whereupon someone else objects. The latter, although warmly dressed, is almost shivering, and cannot bear to have a window open even a bit. The person who is too hot complains, but gives in and accepts his discomfort.

We have all experienced similar problems. In marriage, for instance, the husband is accustomed to sleeping with the windows shut, but his wife cannot possibly fall asleep unless the air she breathes is constantly being renewed.

On public transportation, these different individual responses to the temperature frequently cause arguments. The only rational way of avoiding them is to have a system whereby each individual can regulate the air flow around him. But at present only planes offer their passengers this luxury.

These little everyday problems reflect a fundamental biological truth: the needs of every organism differ. Peter only feels comfortable when the temperature is around 68° F, while Paul prefers the temperature to be about 58° F. One person does not mind breathing air filled with tobacco smoke, while a second person cannot tolerate it. Since none of us lives in isolation, these problems can become frustrating.

Some of these differences can be explained by habits acquired in childhood. Individuals who have had a rugged upbringing are more resistant to the cold than those brought up in a very sheltered environment. Other differences can be attributed to one's native climate. For example, a Congolese arriving in Paris or a Parisian who goes to the Congo are both uncomfortable until they become acclimatized to their new atmospheric environment. Some never become acclimatized. Many Algerians of European descent who came to live in Paris after the Algerian war never adjusted to the Northern European climate. They missed the warm sun of their homeland.

But acquired habits and the climate of one's youth do not explain all individual differences because these differences are found everywhere, even among members of the same family.

Our Personality and Cold Weather

Dr. I. Hoff is concerned with individual differences under the stress of cold weather and has recorded all our physiological reactions when cold. Every individual has a specific blood acidity, calcium-potassium balance, and blood pressure. According to Hoff, these are definitely related to personal reactions of our parasympathetic nervous system. Thus many biometeorologists feel that the type of reaction an individual displays to the weather is closely related both to the subject's physical constitution and to his psychological pattern.

Studies by Doctors B. J. Fine and H. F. Gaydos in 1958

on seventy enlisted men of the United States Army indicated
a number of interesting thermal differences. The subjects
were first subjected to a series of personality tests to determine their psychological differences. Then, clad only in
undershorts, they spent thirty minutes lying in wheelchairs
in a climatic chamber of 70° F, without humidity or wind.
Then the temperature dropped abruptly to 50° F, the room
became humid, and a 5 mph wind blew. These new conditions lasted another thirty minutes. Every subject's temperature was taken at this point, and they were all found to be
several tenths of a degree below normal. A short time later
their temperatures were taken again. The temperature had
returned to normal in those subjects whose character tests
had shown a balanced personality. However, if the personality pattern deviated widely from the norm, the rise in
temperature after the cold exposure took much longer. In
some extreme cases the temperature took twice as long to
return to normal.[20]

Another interesting observation is the importance of body
build. Overweight men feel the cold less than thin men.
However, thin men are more adaptable; they readjust quickly
to the warmth. And if exposure to the cold is prolonged,
thin men suffer less cumulative effects of cold stress than
overweight men.

The Afrikakorps Soldiers

Any person whose body build is very extreme (*i.e.* too
large, too small, too fat, or too thin) is usually less adaptable
to weather changes than a man of normal constitution. Dr.

20. B. J. Fine and H. F. Gaydos, "Relationship between Individual
Personality Variables and Body Temperature Response Patterns in the
Cold" (*Technical Report*, Quartermaster Research Eng. Center, March,
1959).

K. Hoehne proved this assertion in his thesis on the soldiers of the famous Afrikakorps. This group of men, commanded by Field Marshal Erwin Rommel, was engaged in long and fierce fighting against the British during World War II.

The adaptation of these German soldiers to the African climate posed many problems. How could the army chiefs determine which of these Nordic men would acclimatize best? They thought at first that thin, athletic men would be the most adaptable. But this was not the case, even though they did adapt better than corpulent men. The soldiers who adapted most easily were those with the most "average" body builds. Hoehne concluded his study by emphasizing that this confirms a biological axiom: Any exaggerated characteristics of an organism decrease its ability to adapt to new situations. This also confirms the old adage that to be well adapted to one's environment one should not deviate too far from the norm.[21]

Types of Response to Weather

It is well known that certain personality types are predisposed to certain diseases. Rheumatic patients often have an anxious and depressive personality, tubercular patients are very excitable, asthmatics are often hypersensitive, and so on.

These of course are empirical statements. The desire to classify man scientifically according to his response to various kinds of weather is an old dream in medicine. Twenty-five centuries ago Hippocrates was the first to establish such a classification. In his opinion there are four fundamental human types: bilious, sanguineous, nervous, and lymphatic.

21. K. Hoehne: "Konstitution und Reaktionstypen in der Bioklimatik," *Med. Meteorol.*, Vol. 5, no. 66 (1951).

Each type reacts differently to the weather. Later Galen, another famous Greek physician, wrote of the relationship between atmospheric conditions and the physiological and pathological personality of individuals in his treatise "On Temperaments and Humors."

Hippocrates' classification is still accepted today by some doctors. But in the last century a large number of other classifications have been proposed by doctors and psychologists. None has been completely accepted.

Manfred Curry, an American meteorologist living in Germany, developed a new classification some time ago that provoked vehement attacks and defenses by the experts.[22] Curry classified people into two groups according to their reaction to the weather: the K (cold-front)-type and the W(warm-front)-type.*

The typical K-types are introverted and intellectual. Physically, they are slender with long, narrow faces. Their personalities are defensive rather than aggressive. These people, Curry maintains, are very sensitive to the influx of cold air and cold fronts.

The typical W-types are active, dynamic extroverts whose interests center on the outside world with its joys and difficulties. They tend to be solidly built with short, heavy limbs and round faces. They are particularly sensitive to warm fronts and rises in temperature.

Curry's work, along with the enormous amount of material he accumulated, has received considerable attention from doctors. He has made a courageous effort to clarify a difficult problem, but his classification is rather elementary and has not fulfilled the hopes of some physicians.

---

22. M. Curry, *Bioklimatik* (Riederau, 1946).
* K as in *Kaltfront* (cold front); W as in *Warmfront* (warm front).

Meteorosensitive or Meteorostable

Whatever the explanation, it has been established that some people are "sensitive to the weather" and others are not. Weather-sensitive persons become indisposed at the slightest change of weather, while the others cheerfully accept the worst climatic conditions. Mouriquand named the former group "meteorosensitive" and the latter "meteorostable," but as yet no one has been able to provide a good description of the characteristic traits of these two groups.

Weather sensitivity can change in the course of an individual's life. The adaptation curve alters with age. As a general rule, infants are very sensitive, adolescents and adults less so, and elderly people become extremely "meteorosensitive" again.

Intellectual individuals seem very sensitive to cold, heat, and atmospheric turbulence.

Duhot cites the example of one of his patients who always experienced cardiac palpitations and anxiety whenever a storm was approaching. If he was driving at the time, he would have to stop his car and sit by the roadside until the first drops of rain began to fall and brought relief from his symptoms.

De Rudder is of the opinion that difficulty in adapting to weather changes is just one manifestation of a generally temperamental disposition which has difficulty adapting to all changes in life: social-level, familial, and professional changes. According to him, it is easy to recognize "meteorosensitive" people because they are quick to react. They are very emotional and change color rapidly when annoyed. They perspire easily and rarely "feel well."

Evidence

Most great artists, poets and writers are "meteorolabile." They are extremely responsive to their surroundings and have often referred to their own weather sensitivity.

Goethe, the great German poet, was hypersensitive to the weather. Changes of barometric pressure had a strong influence on him. Toward the end of his life, he would always carry a barometer with him in order to foresee what indispositions he risked suffering.

The French novelist Marcel Proust could not tolerate weather changes. We know that he used to have serious asthma attacks, which became much more critical when the weather was changing.

And Madame de Sévigné wrote: "I suffocate three days before a storm; in dry weather my blood seems to dry up in my veins; I am languid when it snows; an indescribable malaise grips me when the sun goes down beyond the horizon. In autumn I become detached from life like a leaf from a tree; and my blood boils in my veins like the sap of a plant when the first rays of the March sun peep through the ceiling of gray clouds." [23]

When Nietzsche, the famous German philosopher, used to travel, he always checked the temperature, barometric pressure, and humidity. Stefan Zweig, his biographer, wrote: "There may never have been an intellectual so sensitive to atmospheric conditions, or so acutely vulnerable to all the variations of meteorological phenomena. His whole body is a pressure gauge. He is a living barometer. He is irritability itself. There seem to be occult electrical impulses between his pulse and the atmospheric pressure, between his nerves and the amount of humidity in the air."

The French philosopher Maine de Biran, wrote numerous

23. Duhot, *op. cit.*, p. 71.

pages in his personal diary from 1792 to 1817 about the relationship between the poor condition of his body and the weather. A human barometer, he felt transformed by every season. "There is no atmospheric change, no matter how slight, which escapes my sensitive system," he wrote.

These examples are sufficient to illustrate the point made above. Weather sensitivity is a reflection of our sensitivity to life itself. If we are easily moved emotionally, then we suffer more—both physically and mentally—from nature's caprices.

THE CYCLE OF SEASONS

Bizarre metamorphoses take place in our bodies during the course of a year. In winter our organs function somewhat differently from the way they function in summer. For example, in summer our hearts beat much faster. This accelerated pace is necessary because our body temperatures rise when the weather is warmer.

Our hair and our beards do not grow at the same rate every season. Eaton, a physiologist, patiently measured the various speeds. Minimum growth occurs in January, when beards grow only about 0.305 millimeters per day. The growth rate accelerates, reaching 0.533 mm. per day in July, 0.538 mm. per day in August, and 0.545 mm. per day in September, the latter figure representing the maximum growth rate. Then it decreases to 0.375 mm. per day in December. So hair grows almost twice as fast in summer as it does in winter.

In healthy individuals the activity of the thyroid gland is at its maximum in spring. This activity decreases in autumn and becomes even more reduced in winter.

Almost all of our bodily systems experience seasonal variations. William Petersen, for example, proved that the blood's pH (acidity level) is at its lowest in April and at its highest in summer. Similarly P. Renbourn found that in summer our hemoglobin level is highest, the red-blood-cell sedimentation rate is fastest, and blood chloride is at its greatest level. In a recent study two French doctors, A. Reinberg and J. Ghata, observed that the excretion of potassium definitely increases in spring, even though no additional amounts of this substance are ingested. This fact leads us to believe that man's adrenal cortex is more active during this season.[1]

We can affirm that *all* functions are actually modified in the course of a year. There are tables in the appendix that illustrate this. These modifications either are caused directly by the season or are an indirect result of seasonal change, related to the fact that the seasons influence our way of life, our diet, and our leisure hours. Thus seasonal changes have many influences on man, affecting his health, birth, well-being, and death.

Winter, a Perilous Season

The link between season and disease has been known since antiquity. Hippocrates was already aware of it when he wrote in his treatise "On Airs, Waters and Places": "Whoever wishes to pursue the science of medicine properly must proceed thus: first he ought to consider what effect each season of the year can produce, for the seasons are not alike but differ widely both in themselves and at their changes." Because of their geographic location, the countries in the temperate zones have four distinct seasons. The days are of variable length. In winter there are fewer hours of daylight than in summer. The average temperature ranges from below freezing in January to the upper seventies in July. It rains more often in spring and autumn than during the rest of the year, but there are more storms in summer, and of course in winter there is snow.

1. A. Reinberg and J. Ghata, *Rythmes et cycles biologiques* (P.U.F., 1957), p. 90.

Studies have shown that winter is definitely the "bad season," the season with the greatest mortality. January, February, and March are the months in which the most deaths occur, regardless of cause. Winter, with its persistent coldness and fog, has always been dreaded by persons with delicate health. It is a generally acknowledged fact in medicine that diseases *a frigore* (*i.e.*, related to the cold weather) are among the most dreaded. But the high mortality rate in winter is also asociated with extremes of age. Thus infants and the elderly are its most frequent victims.

The severer the winter, the greater its death toll. The winter of 1963 was one of the coldest winters in France since the turn of the century. In the report *La Santé et l'Hiver 1963* (Health and the Winter of 1963) made by the National Institute of Hygiene, Marcel Moine states that mortality among persons over sixty years old that winter increased 15.7 percent over the previous winter.

Respiratory diseases strike frequently and severely every year in January, February, and March. So it is in these months that influenza, pneumonia, and bronchopneumonia are most prevalent. Even diseases with no apparent seasonal associations, such as cancer, cirrhosis, or diabetes, cause more deaths during the winter months than during the rest of the year. This is because the cold winter weather adds stress to organs already debilitated from pre-existing disease.

Fatal for Cardiac Patients

Studies by a number of authors clearly indicate that winter is a dangerous season for patients with cardiovascular diseases. In France mortality from cardiac diseases is 30 percent higher in January and February than it is in August and September. I asked a cardiologist the reason for this. "We must correct a common delusion," he said. "For persons with coronary or circulatory diseases, it is the winter, not the summer, that is more harmful, even though both extremes of temperature are dangerous for these patients. In France the temperature rarely reaches a dangerous level in summer, but the patient obviously should be careful not to expose himself to the heat of the sun. This precaution is usually sufficient in summer. In winter, however, it is not rare for temperatures to drop below freezing. Then cardiac patients and persons with high blood pressure are in danger of additional heart strain, especially when the cold weather is accompanied by rain, snow, or an icy wind. This is common medical knowledge. More often than not, the first time I will see a new patient will be in December, January, or February." Paris hospitals report that the number of admissions for cardiovascular disease almost doubles in winter, and other statistical studies completely confirm medical observations in this respect.

Extreme Temperatures

Other major studies made in various parts of the world on cardiac and vascular diseases have reached the same conclusions. At the University of Pennsylvania Drs. Wood and Hedley studied the distribution of coronary thrombosis over a period of three years. Coronary thrombosis is the occlusion of one of the coronary arteries of the heart by the formation of a blood clot. The doctors found that in each of the three years there were many more attacks in autumn and winter, fewer in spring and summer, with a clear minimum during June.

A study of 27,390 cases of angina pectoris by the Bureau of the Census in Washington, D.C., showed a similar seasonal curve. In Germany S. Koller at the statistical department of Bad Nauheim had the patience to record the death dates of

1,600,000 victims of circulatory ailments. His study revealed a clear maximum of deaths in January and February with a minimum in July. Tromp in the Netherlands also made a very complete study of mortality from angina pectoris, coronary thrombosis, cerebral hemorrhage, and myocardial infarction over a period of several years. His results showed that the colder the weather, the greater the number of fatalities from these diseases; and the warmer the weather, the lower the mortality rate.

However, extremely hot weather is as dangerous as cold weather in those parts of the world that are close to the equator. So seasons alone are not the only influential factor. Climate also plays a role. For example, studies by H. E. Heyer and his associates in Dallas, Texas, where the summers are very hot, showed a different clinical picture. It was found that acute myocardial infarction in Texas is more frequent during the hottest season of the year, *i.e.*, during July and August, with maximum temperatures often exceeding 100° F. However, during the rather mild winters in Texas, the incidence of cardiac and vascular disease is low.[2]

Mechanisms Involved

Why do intense heat and severe cold have similar effects on the circulatory system of persons predisposed to or affected with vascular diseases? Doctors believe that the explanation is that these patients have a dysfunction of their thermoregulation mechanism. According to Tromp, heart attacks can be precipitated by several causes. There may be poor functioning of the autonomic nervous system, or there may be changes in the physico-chemical state of the blood.

2. H. E. Heyer and associates, "The increased frequency of acute myocardial infarction during summer months in warm climate," *Am. Heart J.*, Vol. 45, no. 741 (1953).

During the cold winter months blood sedimentation rates are lower, but coagulation time is faster. This can cause an infarction. It seems also that the capillaries are more fragile when the weather is very cold. This would explain the higher incidence of cerebral vascular diseases in winter. High capillary fragility, for example, seems to be the cause of cerebral vascular disease in newborn infants during winter, but fortunately this serious disease is very rare in children born in temperate climates.

Avoiding the Attack

All these observations allow doctors to give some precautionary advice to patients suffering from a weak heart or arteriosclerosis. They must avoid exposure to the cold in winter and to the sun in summer. If possible, at least during the very cold or very hot months, these patients should try to live in areas with mild climates where changes of weather are infrequent. If this is not possible either for professional or financial reasons, they should keep their homes well heated in winter and remain indoors during severe cold spells, on very windy days, and when sudden cold fronts are passing.

Cardiac patients are advised to avoid emotional upsets and strenuous or prolonged physical effort. But this in itself is not enough. Some moderate physical activities, such as walking or gardening, for example, are much less harmful than exposure to the stress of cold or hot weather, because the heat or cold strikes the organism where it is most vulnerable. Popular expressions reflect this idea intuitively. We say, for example, that "the cold hits us" or that "the heat is stifling." A healthy body overcomes the effects of this aggression. But the sickly or highly sensitive organism risks being overwhelmed, sometimes fatally. In his *Biometeorology* Tromp emphasizes the assistance that weather forecasting can offer these cardiac patients. "The population should gradually be educated on these matters by television or radio because this could prolong the life expectancy of numerous cardiac patients. If they were warned in time of the approach of a harmful atmospheric phenomenon, they could take the necessary precautions to avoid its detrimental effects."

Springtime and Tuberculosis

With the advent of antibiotics, tuberculosis is no longer a major cause of death in the Western world, but it is interesting to note that it is a disease very much affected by seasonal changes. The director of a Swiss sanatorium once made the following remark: "If there is one season that worries us more than all the others, it is the spring, for there is a tremendous increase in the incidence of tuberculosis in spring." Not only does the number of tuberculosis patients augment, but there is often the threat of complications, especially hemoptysis. It is in the spring, after long remissions, that relapses tend to occur, and these relapses are often critical.

A detailed study made by Dr. N. J. Strandgaard, a Scandinavian, confirms this observation. His study shows that the results of sanatorium treatment are least satisfactory in spring, whereas the best results are usually obtained in summer and autumn.[3] For the same reason, another physician, Dr. Ernst, strongly advises against operating on tuberculosis patients in spring.

De Rudder reported that in all northern countries of the Northern Hemisphere tuberculosis mortality increases in April and May. Pulmonary tuberculosis is not the only form

3. N. J. Strandgaard, "Seasonal Variation of the Weight of Tuberculosis Patients," *Acta Med. Scand.*, Vol. 57, no. 275 (1923).

of the disease to have a higher incidence in spring. Mortality from tubercular meningitis, for example, is three times higher in spring than in late summer.

There is no convincing explanation for this increased seasonal incidence. Perhaps the bacillus is more virulent in spring; perhaps the individual is more susceptible after the winter and therefore offers less resistance to the bacillus. We do not know. However, K. Ossoinig did observe one interesting fact: namely, that individuals do show seasonal variations in their sensitivity to tuberculin skin tests. They have increased sensitivity in March and April and low sensitivity in autumn.[4] Similar observations were made by Karczag, Amburger, and Peyrer.

In winter the entire organism functions slowly. But in spring it becomes more active. This fact could perhaps be the reason that infections due to Koch's bacillus appear.

Suicides in the Month of May

When the first warm days come, we all feel a desire to escape or run away. It becomes difficult to concentrate on serious matters, and we experience indefinable, vague yearnings that disturb our psychic balance and have a bad influence on our professional activities.

Spring is a period when new romances start, when fresh plans are made, when more marriages take place. But it is also a season when people experience frequent changes of mood and have bitter arguments with one another.

Springtime is a period of both physical and mental effervescence. Duhot has termed this phenomenon the "spring hormonal crisis." The endocrine glands become more active, and consequently sexual activity, in particular, increases. The

4. K. Ossoinig, "Ueber Schwankungen der Tuberculinemfindlichkeit," *Monatsschr. Kinderheilk,* Vol. 31, no. 371 (1926).

endocrine glands are also closely associated with our behavior and mental state. Thus the long-awaited spring is a dangerous season, and the poet's "merry month of May" can often be a very critical month from a psychological point of view.

Fifty years ago Emile Durkheim, a French sociologist, had already pointed out that the greatest number of suicides do not occur in winter or autumn, but in spring, when the beautiful weather comes, when nature smiles, and when temperatures are pleasant. We have only to read the newspapers to confirm that the number of attempted suicides increases with the arrival of the nice weather.

According to psychiatrists, spring is the season when the potentially suicidal subject finally decides to accomplish the fatal act. He buys the lethal poison or opens the gas jets. As a result of the physiological changes it causes in the organism, spring seems to push the desperate toward that final act.

The suicide rate throughout the year follows a specific rhythm with metronomic regularity. Table I which tabulates data from the U.S. Department of Health, Education, and Welfare concerning the number of suicides per month in the United States from 1962 to 1966, illustrates this rhythm. The graph (Figure II) was compiled from these statistics. It shows a systematic fluctuation in the number of suicides in the course of a year. It can be argued that the act of suicide is a free act, but these statistics show that it is strongly determined by seasonal factors. The high frequency of suicides invariably corresponds to the arrival of spring, and this frequency decreases as autumn approaches.

William Petersen, an American biometeorologist, made an interesting discovery. He found that there is another rhythm that is superimposed on the annual suicide rhythm. This second rhythm is determined by the weight and build of the suicidal person. Tall, thin people tend to commit suicide at the beginning of spring. Heavy, stocky individuals wait a few months and tend to choose the beginning of summer. Petersen concluded that men react differently according to their constitution. Thinner people react earlier than heavy individuals to the bad effects of spring.[5]

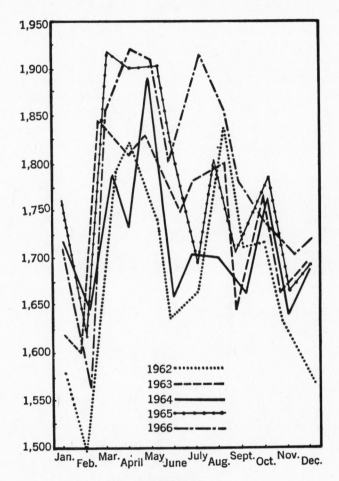

FIGURE II
FLUCTUATIONS IN THE NUMBER OF SUICIDES
PER MONTH DURING THE YEAR

Every year it is in spring that there are the greatest number of suicides and in winter that there are the least. (Based on Table I.)

5. William Petersen, *The Patient and the Weather*, Vol. III (1934), p. 50.

TABLE I

Number of suicides in the United States according to the month of the year

From 1962 to 1966

Year	Jan.	Feb.	Mar.	Apr.	May	June	July	Aug.	Sept.	Oct.	Nov.	Dec.
1962	1583	1499	1787	1824	1738	1636	1659	1838	1713	1721	1636	1573
1963	1621	1601	1849	1817	1831	1750	1782	1801	1645	1769	1664	1695
1964	1717	1647	1785	1735	1889	1661	1706	1702	1659	1758	1639	1690
1965	1757	1620	1921	1903	1904	1825	1698	1805	1711	1783	1665	1689
1966	1714	1568	1861	1924	1914	1801	1917	1855	1781	1738	1710	1724
Total	8392	7935	9203	9203	9276	8673	8762	9001	8509	8769	8314	8371

The Effect on Mental Patients

Psychiatric nurses dread the arrival of spring weather. For them the springtime is a nightmare. Their patients are restless and can become dangerous. They require constant medical surveillance; but this becomes more difficult to provide, since this is the season of the year when institutions are overloaded by the admissions of new patients.

This fact is not new. At the beginning of the eighteenth century a French psychiatrist, Esquirol, observed that the number of mental patient admissions in Paris rose from 162 in January to 265 in July and then decreased again. Dr. C. Willmann's recent study of 13,500 patients in Heidelberg showed a similar curve. Spring restlessness in mental patients is most marked in young patients between the ages of 15 and 30 years

More Crime

The crime rate also increases during the spring. Police officers can verify this from their own daily experience. For example, most cases of kidnapping by mentally deranged persons occur during this season. Women whose maternal love has been frustrated by the lack of children become much more distressed in spring. One psychiatric report mentioned the case of a fifty-year-old woman who was of normal intelligence and from a good family. But every year when the spring weather arrived and the public parks were once again filled with the happy laughter of children, she would have an overwhelming desire to run off with a baby carriage and push it along in front of her for hours and hours.

Paradoxically, there are also more child murders at this time of year. In Freiburg, Germany, U. Westphal observed a definite increase in the number of infanticides during the spring. Also in Germany, O. Bumke undertook a detailed study of sexual offenses. The graph of his results forms a curve similar to the one obtained for the monthly suicide rate. Taking an average rate of 100 sexual offenses per month, the maximum number (152) occurs during March, April, and May and the minimum (65) occurs during September, October, and November.

The sexual activity of normal people follows a similar rhythm. Doctor W. Otto [6] has gathered some interesting statistics in this respect. In Northern Europe most illegitimate conceptions occur in May, while most legitimate conceptions occur one or two months later. This fact seems to indicate that spring may very well be the season for all forms of impulsive behavior.

Hay Fever

In June, instead of taking advantage of the long, sunny days, many people have to stay indoors because of a very unpleasant indisposition, hay fever, or pollinosis, as it is called medically. This is a very distressing complaint. The patient's nose runs constantly, and he sneezes excessively. His nose, mouth, and pharynx itch. His sinuses may become obstructed, and this can precipitate severe headaches.

Hay fever is an allergy caused by the pollen of various plants. The term "hay fever" is actually incorrect, because the clinical symptoms are never caused by hay but by pollen allergens produced by plants usually flowering around the hay-making season.

6. W. Otto, *Jahreszeitliche Vorteilung von Lebendgebotenen, Früh-geborenen, Totgeborenen und Gestorbenen, Arztl. Forsch.* Vol. no. 14, no. 40 (1960).

Hay-fever symptoms unassociated with seasonal phenomena may be caused by house dust, fresh paint, decorating materials, or even a pillow containing allergens.

It is in summer that hay fever becomes prevalent, and here meteorological factors play a considerable role because they control the amount of pollen and spores in the air. On sunny days wind serves to carry the pollen far and wide. But when it rains, the pollen is washed to the ground, and so the air is cleared and relief is brought to the allergy sufferers.

Cooke, an American, listed the following allergy-provoking pollens. In early spring tree pollens are the worst offenders, especially pollen from elm, poplar, ash, beech, oak, and birch (in this order of appearance). During May and June grasses start pollinating and provoking allergies—in particular meadow grass, darnel, barley, fescue, and plantain. The fall type of hay fever is caused chiefly by ragweed.

The allergenic role of these pollens has been proved by giving skin tests using extracts of the pollens believed responsible for producing the allergic symptoms. Redness and local irritation can be seen in allergic persons where the test was applied.

Overrun by Ragweed

The primary cause of 90 percent of hay fever is a weed known as ragweed, which pollinates from mid-August to first frost. Ragweed is a leafy plant ranging in length from twelve to sixty inches. It has furry stems with deeply lobed or dissected leaves and long spikes of greenish-yellow flowers. It produces enormous amounts of pollen, which is disseminated by wind. In one season it can produce more than a billion pollen grains, or about eight million grains in five hours. Every summer it victimizes many thousands of peo ple. In New York state alone more than one million people suffer from ragweed allergies that sometimes force them to stop work temporarily.

Ragweed was brought to Europe by American troops during World War II, and it has since proliferated along the sides of the roads that they traveled. It did not seem to spread any further for a long time. Then in 1966 the situation began to change, and ragweed started gaining ground. This change is attributed to the many construction projects that dug up the soil, leaving the earth exposed for ragweed seeding. Also the building of new roads has been particularly conducive to the spread of ragweed. The sides of the roads where the soil has recently been disturbed and then not replanted with any grass have encouraged the proliferation of ragweed.

Poliomyelitis, a Summer Catastrophe

It is now summer. Man has managed to survive the crisis of spring, but already other dangers await him. First among them in the United States used to be the dreaded disease poliomyelitis. This summer and end-of-summer disease used to leave many children debilitated for the rest of their lives. Now, however, it has been conquered in the United States by vaccines developed in America by Drs. Salk and Sabin and by Professor Lépine in France. *The New York Times* reported on July 7, 1970, that there was not a single death from poliomyelitis in the United States in 1969 and that there were only 19 cases of paralytic poliomyelitis in the entire country. But poliomyelitis has not yet been completely eliminated—far from it. It can even strike adults. Doctors and parents should always be mindful that summer is a dangerous season for this illness. Influenza symptoms in summer are a warning signal that medical advice should be sought to verify that the patient does not have poliomyelitis.

All health authorities agree that mortality from poliomyelitis increases during the summer months. The National Institute of Hygiene in France conducted a study on deaths from poliomyelitis from 1954 to 1961. Every year they found that the mortality rate was higher in July and August—which is the time when poliomyelitis is three times more prevalent—than during the other months of the year.

This same seasonal rhythm has been observed in other countries too. In Germany, where poliomyelitis has been the subject of many investigations, Dr. Wernstadt found that 64.6 percent of the cases occur in summer as opposed to 35.4 percent in winter. De Rudder has proven that during years when there have been epidemics, the incidence of poliomyelitis is fifty times higher in summer than in winter.

A Disease of Clean Countries

Most serious infectious diseases such as cholera, dysentery, and typhoid fever strike in the summer. The heat coupled with unhygienic conditions favors the dissemination of these diseases. However, today they are prevalent only in very warm, underdeveloped countries where hygiene still leaves much to be desired. But strange to note, poliomyelitis is an exception to this pattern. Although it too is an infectious disease, it is not commonly prevalent in warm, underdeveloped countries. The farther a country lies from the equator, the more frequently and more violently poliomyelitis seems to occur. For example, epidemics in Scandinavia are usually more violent than those in Germany, which in turn are more violent than those in Italy; finally, there are relatively few serious cases in Africa, where the virus does exist although it does not cause paralysis. Paradoxically, and unlike other infectious diseases, poliomyelitis is a disease of "clean people." More than proper hygiene is needed to combat it.

How does a poliomyelitis epidemic originate? We know that the filterable poliomyelitis virus is transmitted by direct contact with the virus carrier. It enters through the upper airways (*i.e.*, the nose, pharynx, or tonsils). It can also be acquired from water. Certain meteorological conditions seem to lower the local resistance to the poliomyelitis virus in the respiratory tract. In the opinion of Dr. Armstrong, Director of the Microbiological Institute in Bethesda, Maryland, humidity is a determining factor. During a poliomyelitis epidemic in the United States he noticed that the virus was able to penetrate the body's mucous membranes more easily in warm and humid weather. Yet rain itself is not a cause. Doctor E. Rethly, who studied epidemics in Hungary from 1931 to 1947, observed that these epidemics did not occur more frequently during wet years.

Kling's theory states that poliomyelitis is caught mainly near water: near coasts, lakes, and rivers. It is a fact that many epidemics follow the course of rivers. Formerly it was believed that viruses were transported by the water. But this theory has since been rejected because studies have shown that epidemics occasionally follow the river's course upstream, as happened, for example, along the Rhine during the severe 1927 epidemic in Alsace.

Although we do not know how viruses are propagated, there seems to be general agreement that a large concentration of individual carriers of the viruses is definitely a major factor involved in creating an epidemic. Large numbers of people living in the same locality are conducive to epidemics. Furthermore, many large cities are located near rivers or large bodies of water. It is apparent that rivers are contaminated by human excretion harboring the virus, hence these bodies of water have been associated with epidemics. But as we have seen, the path taken by the epidemic is not always the same as the river's course. It more often follows the direction taken by the individual carriers of the virus.

Seasonal Pediatric Illnesses

Infantile mortality rates when examined in relation to the four seasons show a sudden increase during August and September. One of the contributing causes of this late-summer increase is gastroenteritis. During the very warm summer months young infants risk catching an infection from milk that has not been properly sterilized.

Until 1913, 36 percent of infant mortalities in summer were caused by gastroenteritis, according to figures from the National Institute of Statistics. Fortunately this mortality rate has been lowered thanks to new methods of treatment and stricter control of the purity of milk. Today gastroenteritis is responsible for only 12 percent of infant mortalities.

But this figure is still too high. Parents should be doubly careful in summer with regard to the food they give their infants and young children.

Even in the healthiest child there is a constant conflict between his fragile body and harmful bacteria. It is in autumn, when the child is starting school, that this conflict becomes most acute. Who has not been as a child exposed to whooping cough and measles, scarlet fever, and chicken pox? Some of these pediatric diseases are unpleasant, but benign. Others are very serious. The most dangerous of all are undoubtedly diphtheria and cerebro-spinal meningitis, two diseases that become prevalent as winter approaches.

Diphtheria is the first to strike. It makes its appearance in October. Then it is followed by cerebro-spinal meningitis, which reaches its period of maximum incidence during February and March. Whooping cough and scarlet fever epidemics generally occur toward the end of winter in March. And finally, measles, which is the commonest childhood disease, is quite rare at the beginning of winter but becomes prevalent from April to July. Figure III shows the seasonal variations of these pediatric diseases.

Fortunately, diphtheria, whooping cough, and measles can now all be prevented by inoculation; and for reasons unknown scarlet fever has become a much milder disease

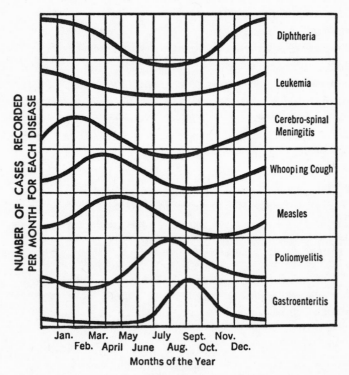

NUMBER OF CASES RECORDED PER MONTH FOR EACH DISEASE

Diphtheria

Leukemia

Cerebro-spinal Meningitis

Whooping Cough

Measles

Poliomyelitis

Gastroenteritis

Jan.   Mar.   May   July   Sept.   Nov.
  Feb.   April   June   Aug.   Oct.   Dec.
Months of the Year

FIGURE III
SEASONAL VARIATIONS OF SOME PEDIATRIC DISEASES

Each disease has a somewhat different periodicity. Only poliomyelitis and gastroenteritis strike in midsummer. (From the documentation of the National Institute of Statistics & Economics and the National Institute of Hygiene, and the Cancer Journal.)

than it used to be, and in any event can be quickly cured with penicillin.

Identical seasonal variations occur in the United States and in all countries in Europe. Numerous studies have confirmed these seasonal variations on both continents.

Seasonal Incidence of Leukemia

In the acute variety most of leukemia's victims are children. Very little is known yet about this deadly disease, but pending further knowledge, it may be regarded as a "cancer of the blood," because the blood of leukemic patients reveals an abnormal increase in the number of white blood cells and an invasion by vast numbers of embryonic cells called leukoblasts. There is excessive production of white blood cells in the bone marrow, which no longer functions properly and has lost its ability to prevent the proliferation of abnormal and harmful cells. The patient soon starts showing visible symptoms of the disease: pallor, exhaustion, headaches, frequent hemorrhages, fever, enlarged spleen and liver. Though death can sometimes be delayed, no cure has yet been found.

Studies show that, surprisingly, the first symptoms of acute leukemia generally appear in winter, rarely in summer. This has been confirmed by many doctors—Drs. Lambin and Gérard in Belgium, Dr. Scanu in Rome and Naples, and Dr. Gerola in Northern Italy, to mention a few. In the United States a very extensive study involving thousands of cases was performed by Donald H. Hayes at the North Carolina Baptist Hospital. He found that acute leukemia has its onset with greatest frequency between December and April and with lowest frequency during August and September.[7]

7. D. H. Hayes: "The Seasonal Incidence of Acute Leukemia," *Cancer* (1960), 14, 1301, 19.

No explanation has yet been found for this phenomenon. Doctors have accepted the facts and are trying to find the reason. Some viral diseases—influenza, for example—are also more prevalent in winter. This parallel has led to the suggestion that seasonal variations in the incidence of leukemia may be related to an infectious process that we still know nothing about—a virus, for example. But the seasonal variations can also be explained another way. Both the size and activity of the endocrine glands are subject to seasonal changes. They are larger and given to more active cellular reproduction in late rather than in early winter.

Fertility Rhythms

The frequency of human births follows a very distinct seasonal pattern. Of course, this rhythm can obviously vary from one year to the next as a result of circumstances. A late-winter influenza epidemic alters the annual curve because nine months later there are fewer births. But as a general rule there are more births in late spring and early summer and fewer births in November and December.

Dr. John Meyer found the following number of births in the Lyonnais region in France from 1950 to 1955: spring— 5,927; summer—5,871; autumn—5,099; winter—5530.[8]

The birth rate is at its peak during May. Going back nine months from May places the time of conception in August, which is vacation time for many people. Is the fertility rhythm therefore related to vacation time? asked Doctor Meyer. Vacations do offer unusually beneficial conditions for sexual activity: idleness, warmth, exposed bodies, and more opportunity are all factors to be considered.

In order to find out if birth rhythms are caused by social

8. J. Meyer, *Des Variations saisonnières, mensuelles, quotidiennes et horaires du nombre des accouchements,* medical thesis, Lyon, 1956.

organization, Meyer decided to find out whether the increased incidence of conception in August had been reinforced by the institution of paid summer vacations. In 1925, there was still no such thing in France. But his research showed that even then more children were being conceived in summer.

So there seems to be a genuine seasonal rhythm that is part of our physiology. The condition of the endocrine glands favors reproduction in summer but diminishes reproductive power in winter. Vitamins have an important influence on the functioning of the endocrine glands. Winter causes a vitamin E and C deficiency, which could explain the lower conception rate during this season. Vitamin E is very important for the males of all species. Scientists have discovered that a vitamin E deficiency in male mice slows spermatogenesis and causes irreversible atrophy of the seminiferous tubes.

On the other hand, the pituitary and the corpus luteum in females require large amounts of vitamin C (ascorbic acid). As Dr. Renaud remarked, vitamin C is a progestational compound that is indispensable for procreation and gestation.

Physical Constitution and Month of Birth

The works of Dr. H. Abels in Germany seem to confirm the hormonal theory of seasonal fertility rhythms. He found that babies born in summer were on the average seven ounces heavier at birth than babies born in winter. My own personal research involving several thousand children born in Paris reached similar conclusions. The larger, more robust children seem to be those who are conceived at a time when procreation impulses are the strongest.[9]

9. H. Abels; Ueber die Wichtigkeit der Vitamine für die Entwicklung des Menschlichen fötalen und mütterlichen Organismus *Klin Wschr.*, Vol. 2, no. 1785 (1922).

Other interesting conclusions can be drawn. For example, the birth month of a child can give some indication of his future physical constitution, as several serious studies have shown. Two French authorities, Reinberg and Ghata, have mentioned the studies of an English demographer, Mr. Fitt: "Fitt recently published the results of a study of 21,000 New Zealand soldiers who fought in World War II. The height and weight of every sold:er was recorded. The tallest were born in February and the shortest in June. The heaviest were born in December and the lightest in June. However, the weight differences were relatively less important than the differences in size." [10]

If we evaluate these birth months in terms of the Northern Hemisphere, Fitt's research shows that the tallest people are born in August and the shortest in December. The heaviest individuals are born in June and the lightest in December.

Season and Mental Deficiency

A mentally deficient person is an individual who does not score as well on intelligence tests as a normal subject of the same age. Psychologists consider a subject to be mentally deficient when his intelligence quotient is lower than 70 (the average I.Q. is set at 100). Although the mentally deficient individual may be able to reason, he can solve only very simple problems. He is unable to keep up with the rest of his class in school and ought to be educated in special institutions. Mentally deficient persons are often a burden to their families and to society.

There can be many origins of mental deficiency, and one of these is unquestionably a seasonal factor. Two American

10. A. Reinberg and J. Ghata, *Cycles et rythmes biologiques* (P.U.F.), p. 91.

scientists, H. Knobloch and B. Pasamanick, conducted a study on this question of seasonal influence and found ample support for their theory, which was published in the American Journal of Public Health 1958.[11]

They traced the birth dates of all mentally deficient children admitted to the Columbus State School who were born between 1913 and 1948. They discovered that these children had been born mainly in the winter (see Table II).

For example, 1507 of them were born in February as compared to only 1297 in August. One might think that the difference was due to the bad winter weather, which impeded the child's development during the first few weeks after his birth. But this is not so, according to these investigators. It is the summer heat during the early months of gestation that has a harmful influence on the development of the brain cells. The formation of the cerebral cortex takes place during the third month of pregnancy. Any injury occurring at this time can substantially involve the child's future intellectual functioning.

According to Knobloch and Pasamanick, this is what happens when the first months of pregnancy occur during the hot summer months: The future mother loses her appetite. She has no desire to eat rich, solid food and tends to eat less. Her protein intake may become too low. This decreased dietary intake can hinder the development of the fetal brain at a very critical period.

Heat appears to play a definite role because they found that fewer mentally deficient children have been born when the first ten weeks of pregnancy have occurred during temperate summers than when these weeks have occurred during very hot summers. The authors have provided some convincing statistics. When the first ten weeks of pregnancy corresponded to an exceptionally hot period during July and

11. H. Knobloch and B. Pasamanick, "Seasonal variation in the births of the mentally deficient, *Am. J. Public Health*, Vol. 48, no. 1201 (1958).

August, they found that 3,177 mentally deficient children were born. But during years when cooler temperatures were recorded in July and August, their studies show only 2,482 such listings, which is approximately one-third less.

TABLE II

Number of Mentally Deficient Children Born Each Month
Period from 1913–48

(From Knobloch and Pasamanick, *American Journal of Public Health,* 1958).

Jan.	Feb.	Mar.	Apr.	May	June	Jul.	Aug.	Sept.	Oct.	Nov.	Dec.
1,402	1,507	1,422	1,386	1,385	1,349	1,321	1,297	1,337	1,306	1,416	1,414

The Months for Intelligence

The seasonal, meteorological environment can therefore harm the intellectual development of the fetus during gestation. But this environment can likewise assist intellectual development when circumstances are favorable. Florence Goodenough, an American psychologist, observed that children of school age who had been born in summer had a slightly higher intelligence quotient than those born in winter. Clarence Mills made a similar observation in Cincinnati: children born in summer are twice as likely to pass a college entrance examination as those born in winter.

Another psychologist, J. E. Orme, studied this question in adults. In *The British Journal of Psychology* he explains how he compared two groups of adults.[12] The first group was composed of mental retardates who lived in a special institution. The majority of them had been born in winter. For a second group made up of "supra-normal" subjects, Orme

12. J. E. Orme, "Ability and Season of Birth," *The British Journal of Psychology*, No. 56 (1965), p. 471.

went to Mensa, which was founded in Oxford in 1945. This club is formed exclusively of people with I.Q.s higher than 149 (100 being the I.Q. of a normal individual). Only 10,000 people in the entire world are said to have been made members of this organization. Orme discovered that very few of the "supra-normal" subjects in Mensa were born in winter. He concluded his study by saying: "It seems therefore that temperatures during fetal development are as important for the child's future intelligence as the conditions surrounding his birth or conception."

Other investigators have shown the importance of meteorological conditions during gestation upon the child's future life. For example, some types of cerebral paralysis and epilepsy, some reading defects, tics, and even some behavioral problems may be the belated manifestation of the harmful effect of excessively warm weather during the first weeks of gestation.

A Season for Schizophrenia

A similar clinical picture can be seen in several mental diseases. Schizophrenia, for example, is probably the most serious and the most widespread mental disorder. It begins insidiously and evolves slowly. But the general course of the disease is more or less inevitable. It usually appears in late childhood or adolescence.

Schizophrenia is derived from the Greek and means "splitting of the mind." It is characterized by progressive withdrawal from people and outside activities. Initially the subject's disposition changes. He neglects his family and friends. Then his intellectual functions become impaired. He can no longer make the effort to concentrate. He quits his work. Gradually over the years he becomes more and more demented.

A Dutch psychiatrist, Sauvage Nolting, published in *The Netherlands Journal of Mental Health* the results of a vast study concerning the dates of birth of 2,090 schizophrenics. Six hundred and twenty-eight of these patients had been born in winter (January, February, March) as opposed to only 428 born in summer (July, August, September). The author explains the higher birth rate in winter by a shortage of certain vitamins during gestation. This lack would adversely affect the fetus, which would later show a greater susceptibility than others to schizophrenia.[13]

On the other hand, Petersen's statistics indicate that humanity's greatest geniuses tend to be conceived in April. Is the distance between insanity and genius really so short? Obviously slight statistical tendencies cannot be the basis for fixed rules. As Reinberg and Ghata appropriately commented, "We do not feel that we can advise couples who would like to give birth to a future genius to procreate in April. They could be disappointed because statistics show that the number of mentally retarded born in winter is proportionally much greater than the number of geniuses."

Eugenic Advice?

Fitt spent his life studying these problems. He has examined muscular capacity, mental capacity, frequency of pediatric diseases, juvenile delinquency, and suicidal tendencies in relation to the month of conception. He now has no doubt that conceptions occurring in spring or summer are less favorable because the mother and her future child risk suffering stresses that are more harmful than at other times of the year. In his opinion children conceived in spring or summer tend to have subsequent pathology.

13. Sauvage Nolting, "Relation between Month of Birth and Schizophrenia, *Ned. Tijdschr,* Geneesk 95, 3855 (1951).

However, the parents of children who, for example, were conceived in May and born in February should not be unduly alarmed. The studies cited are only statistical results. The great majority of winter births yield and will continue to yield fine children who grow up to be healthy, well-balanced adults.

But the statistics quoted above do contain an important message. The pregnant mother should be careful to follow a diet that will be beneficial to the development of her future child. If the child is conceived during a period of stress, she should take some special precautions to see that her diet is adequate in vitamins and protein, because the future physical and mental health of her child is at stake. She should also consult her physician regularly during pregnancy. He alone can determine if the mother, and consequently the child she is carrying, are suffering from any dietary deficiencies.

In the light of the tendencies presented above, should parents be given advice on eugenics? Should they, for example, be advised against conceiving children in spring and summer? This would be much too premature. First, we cannot predict the weather for any given year. And second, scientists are far from understanding the physiological mechanisms of pregnancy and their relationship to the environment. A balanced diet and careful hygiene are definitely more important than all other factors.

Round the Clock

The alternation between day and night makes every day a miniature year. Every day consists of four smaller intervals that we call morning, afternoon, evening, and night. These daily divisions are 365 times shorter than the four annual seasons. But, on the other hand, they occur 365 times more frequently. And so this daily rhythm causes modifications within the annual rhythm of our lives.

The consequences of this daily rhythm are truly considerable, as is evidenced by the large number of scientific papers published on this topic. Scientists have called this rhythm established by the constant alternation of day and night the "diurnal rhythm."

Every meteorological factor varies in the course of a day, and man is affected by these changes. Even the strongest wind abates in the evening. During the twenty-four hours of the day, light, temperature, humidity, and atmospheric pressure undergo significant variations that are felt by our bodies. Storms, for example, occur more frequently during late afternoon because there is more electricity in the air at this time.

Our waking-sleeping cycle is dependent on the alternation of day and night. Activity during the day and rest at night modify the body's state. The blood pressure and body temperature of a healthy individual are higher in the evening than in the early hours of the morning. All our bodily functions vary during the course of a day. In the opinion of F. Halberg, an American biologist, "A man is not the same person at 10 A.M. as at 10 P.M."

From the moment we are born, we are bound to this daily rhythm. The staffs of obstetric clinics are quite used to having a host of deliveries every night around the same time. Babies tend to be born in the early hours of the morning (unless, of course, the physician is inducing delivery). This is because the mother generally experiences her first labor pains around midnight. Fatigued at the end of the day, she relaxes during her first deep sleep, and this muscular relaxation allows labor to commence. And so, as Dr. J. Malek from Prague has proved, it is easier for a woman to give birth at night than during the day. The delivery is faster, easier, and less painful.[14]

14. J. Malek and associates: "Characteristics of Daily Rhythm of Menstruation and Labor" (*Ann. of the N.Y. Acad. of Sciences*, 98, 142, 1962).

Birth is not the only aspect of our lives to be related to the daily environment. All our comfort and pain depend on it. Each of us is familiar with the painful toothache that worsens just as we are trying to fall asleep.

Duhot has pointed out that many diseases tend to become manifest at certain specific times: "Attacks of laryngitis stridulosa (false croup), acute pulmonary edema, asthma attacks, and attacks of gout tend to occur at night. On the other hand, epileptic fits are more frequent during the day." [15]

Even in the book of *Job* it was written that man tends to die in the early hours of the morning. Studies by demographers have confirmed this observation made thousands of years ago. The natural, daily mortality rhythm follows a curve whose peak occurs at approximately 3 to 4 A.M. and whose lowest point occurs at the beginning of the afternoon. The dying person holds onto life for a part of the night, but then, exhausted, he dies. In short, we are born and we die at almost the same time of day.

A Time for Every Medication

Our daily physiological rhythm plays an important role therapeutically, but for many years this role was disregarded. During a conference on "Man's Dependence on the Earthly Atmosphere," F. Halberg emphasized the effect of this diurnal rhythm on the action of various medications. "It is not enough," he declared, "to give the right dose of the right medication. It should also be given *at the right time of day*." [16]

Drugs have different effects according to the time of day they are administered. For example, a certain poison injected

15. Duhot, *op. cit.*, p. 41.
16. F. Halberg: "Physiologic 24 Hour Rhythms," *Man's Dependence on the Earthly Atmosphere* (1962), p. 48.

into a mouse in the morning will kill it, whereas the same dose injected in the evening, will not cause death. It is therefore necessary for the doctor to know the varying action of the medicine he is prescribing, especially when treating cases of shock.

Time of day also plays an influential role in surgical operations. It has been observed that the regeneration of wounded organs differs according to the time of the surgery because very significant variations in the speed of cellular division occur in the course of a day. This is valid not only for the healing process after surgery, but also in the case of malignant tumors. These cancerous growths develop faster at midday than in the morning or evening.

All these factors are very important in medicine. A better knowledge of daily biological rhythms could help us select the best time to take a certain medication, give an injection, or perform an operation by taking into consideration the fluctuations of the disease in the course of a twenty-four-hour period.

Disturbed Biological Clocks

Our cells become so accustomed to the diurnal rhythm of day and night that they eventually take it for granted. One could say that we have a sort of "biological clock" within us.

However, technical progress has violated these clocks. Air travel, for example, risks disturbing their well-regulated functions and asynchronizes the well-established physiological rhythm. A recent issue of the *New York Bulletin of the Academy of Sciences* has described the symptoms of jet-travel sickness caused by long plane trips.

Here is what happened to an American businesman who went to Greece by air. He left New York at 6 P.M. and spent nine hours in the air en route to Athens. When he arrived, it was 9 A.M. there but 3 A.M. in New York. This man had crossed five time zones in less than half a day. When he disembarked from the plane, his body was performing at its lowest physiological level. But there was no question of his taking a rest. Everyone else was at work. He was given a warm welcome. He had to attend a cocktail party, go to a business luncheon, and so on through the day. Then he began to suffer from "asynchronization." The first symptoms of it are fatigue, anxiety, depression, and especially stomach complaints. As Dr. Hubertus Strughold remarked at a conference at the Military Aerospace Academy, it is the stomach, which is very fastidious about its established routine, that suffers most in jet travel.

This businessman, however, had no specific organic attack. He was in excellent health. But his body's biological clock was out of order. The functions dependent on it were no longer coordinated. The biological clock cannot be "set at the correct time" as easily as a wristwatch.

This type of physiological irregularity will no doubt become more critical in future extraterrestrial voyages. In their orbits around the earth, the astronauts see a good many sunrises and sunsets every twenty-four hours. Their physiological adaptation to time can be completely disturbed. Space physicians are very concerned with this important problem. An American biologist, F. A. Brown, even proposed a strange space project that attracted the attention of NASA. In this space voyage the astronaut would be replaced by a potato! If the potato died, this would be a very bad sign for long-duration manned space flights according to Professor Brown.

Why does the potato run the risk of dying? Because the internal clock that regulates its entire metabolism may become disturbed when it is beyond the terrestrial synchronizations that usually regulate it. It will be interesting to see how the first men chosen to live on the moon will adapt to the day-night cycle there which lasts twenty-seven days. Will their bodies be able to adapt to this new rhythmic cycle?

Throughout history man has shown such a remarkable capacity to adapt to the most adverse circumstances that he will almost certainly resolve this new difficulty caused by the disturbance of his biological clock. But only the future will tell us how.

THE RANGE OF CLIMATES

We are accustomed to the climate of the country in which we live. The weather varies daily, seasons change every few months, and climatic influences are constant. "It is remarkable to see to what extent the climate of a country influences not only the civilization of the people inhabiting it, but also their physiology and pathology. This correlation may be direct, as, for instance, the languid influence of a tropical climate or the recurrence of rheumatic and respiratory disease in cold, damp environments. Or the correlation can be indirect, affecting, for example, the growth of certain flora or fauna, which in turn has a characteristic influence on man." [1]

The human race has been molded by the various climates of this planet. Throughout the ages scientists have been struck by how well the inhabitants of a given area have adapted to the particular climate of that region. In the Scandinavian countries the sun is low and often blocked by clouds. The people living there are fair-haired and have pale complexions, sensitive to the sun's weakest rays. Dark-skinned races live on the sunny shores of the Mediterranean, and Negroes are natives of the scorching tropics. As early as elementary school we learn the importance of the brightly colored, contrast-

1. Rivolier, *La Biométéorologie*, p. 5.

ing horizontal bands that encircle the globe. In the center is the equatorial zone with its hot, humid climate. Then there are two tropical desert regions to the north and south of it. These in turn are bordered above and below by the two temperate zones. And finally there are the polar regions, buried in ice, where the cold reigns supreme.

But these climates have not always been what they are today. Climatic upheavals have, in the past, created some civilizations and destroyed others, and they have transformed modes of life on earth. Since time began, and for reasons that are still obscure, there have been extremely warm and extremely cold periods on earth. Traces of the recurrent advance and retreat of glaciers in the temperate zones bear witness to this fact. These climatic changes have affected our whole history. When the European climate was bitterly cold, the present-day deserts were a paradise for man. Then, as the European climate gradually turned milder, the deserts became arid. Soon the people living there were forced to flee. They reached the banks of the Nile and settled there. Thus began the great Egyptian civilization.

Climates are not defined only in terms of their distance from the north and south poles or from the equator. Many other factors play a role. We know that the sea exerts a moderating influence on countries bounded by oceans. The winters are never very cold and the summers are rarely too hot. Western Europe profits from this kind of thermal regulation. Inland, far from the maritime coasts, as in central Asia for example, the climate is harsh and the seasons change abruptly. This severe "continental" climate toughens the inhabitants. The climate of a country is also affected by winds, like the Tyrolian foehn; by rains, such as the monsoons of India; by altitude, as illustrated by the Andes plateaus; and by the number of inhabitants, as in our large modern cities. All these factors influence man's health.

The regional climates of a country are also very important. In France alone there are about ten distinct climates. Rivolier cited a typical example of this regional climatic influence on our health. A small town in Brittany has only eight thousand inhabitants. Yet several ear, nose, and throat specialists are required to serve the people. A town of the same size in the south of France has no such specialists. If a resident has an ear, nose, or throat complaint he must go to another city for treatment. But this does not often happen because the clear, sunny climate in this area is better for the respiratory tract than the Breton climate in the north.

Bacteria and Climate

Bacteria and viruses are also prevalent in certain climates. Through epidemics, climates exert an influence on the general health of countries. Infectious diseases that strike throughout the world do not present the same danger in every latitude. Some scourges that are devastating in one place are barely felt in others, as we have seen in the case of poliomyelitis. This disease becomes more deadly the further it strikes from the equator. There are other serious infectious diseases that are prevalent only in hot countries.

The mechanism of epidemics linked to climate is often very complicated. Let us examine the case of paludism, or malaria as it is commonly called. This infectious disease is characterized by severe chills followed by high fever. Caused by the presence of a parasite, *genus plasmodium,* in the red blood cells, the disease is transmitted by the bite of the anopheles mosquito. There are many anopheles-free, hence malaria-free zones, because plasmodium and the anopheles mosquito only develop in certain specific climates—those with high temperatures and high humidity. But these two climatic conditions alone do not cause a malarial epidemic. The anopheles mosquito must first become infected by biting a person with malaria. It then transmits the disease by biting another person.

Malaria is endemic in lower Egypt, West Africa, Mada-gascar, Indochina, Mexico, and the West Indies. In Europe there are malarial areas in the swamps of southern Russia and in Greece, Spain, and Rumania. Italy was also plagued by the disease until the Pontine Marshes near Rome were drained.

Similar complex factors control the spread of yellow fever in the world. Yellow fever is endemic in certain por-tions of South and Central America and along the African coast (Senegal, Nigeria), where it was imported. Climate favors its spread in these areas because there are virgin forests close to the towns and villages. Man must go into the jungle to be bitten by the mosquito carrying yellow fever.

Man's Role

The human factor superimposes itself on climatic con-ditions. Man transforms nature, and this in turn modifies the climate. He can divert waterways, construct dams, destroy forests, impoverish the soil, pollute the water, and build huge cities.

But man has even greater dreams. Some scientists fore-see irrigating the Sahara desert by tapping the water that has been stored deep within the earth since the formation of the world. Some Soviet engineers would like to close the Bering Straits in Northern Asia, thus altering the winds and rainfall over most of Siberia.

Furthermore, man is itinerant. Since the dawn of history men living in regions with poor soil have been attracted by more fertile areas. Whether as conquering warriors or peace-ful immigrants, they have been forced to adapt to different climates in new lands.

The "visitors" are not the only ones to suffer the effects of relocation. The fate of the "visited" people is often unenviable. Immigrants bring with them diseases that were prevalent in their climate of origin. Many terrible epidemics have been disseminated throughout the ages by infected migrants. Stringent sanitary measures did succeed in minimizing these dangers for a long time. But the extreme ease with which we can travel today from country to country has renewed the menace.

In January 1966, Dr. Claude Bétourné, a physician at a Paris hospital, disclosed that tropical diseases such as malaria, leprosy, and amebiasis were becoming more common in the Paris area. Numerous trips to Africa by Europeans and the large number of workers coming from Africa and the West Indies have brought countless parasitic diseases into the French capital. Thus doctors have been confronted with a new medical problem. The general practitioner must learn to diagnose diseases that he is not accustomed to seeing. Take the case of a champion cyclist from Italy who died several days after a trip to Africa, where he had contracted a deadly form of malaria. His life might been saved if the correct diagnosis of his illness had been made in time. Bétourné brought this problem to the attention of his colleagues in Paris: "If one of your patients, who has just disembarked at Orly airport from Africa, comes to you and complains of chills and has a very high temperature, he may merely have the flu; but he could very well be suffering from something else, a malarial attack for example. Do not wait for him to sink into a coma before you become aware of this possibility."

Cases of sleeping sickness and leprosy have been observed in Negroes from Mali and Mauritania now working in Paris (but these diseases can strike any race). Diseases which are even more infrequent have also been observed recently, for example, hydatid cysts, filariasis and schistosomiasis. As for amebiasis the health centers responsible for analyzing medical statistics have noted a sizable increase of amoebae in the intestines of Parisians over the past twenty years.

Knowledge to Be Discovered

The role climate plays in disease has been studied since Hippocrates. Yet J. M. May, an authority on this subject, notes that very few theories have been confirmed up to the present time. "It is not wise to deviate from the line of what is strictly proved," he wrote, "lest one fall into the realm of folklore." [2]

This is a very strong opinion. However, medical experts have carefully examined the way in which certain climates facilitate the curing of many diseases, and the deleterious effect of other climates on some diseases.

Today we are trying to further this knowledge. Precise studies have provided detailed climatic information regarding such illnesses as the rheumatic diseases, rickets, tuberculosis, and cancer.

Rheumatic Diseases and Cold Countries

The incidence of rheumatism varies from country to country and within each country. The harmful influence of cold, damp climates is obvious. In the United States studies by C. A. Mills have shown that there are five times more rheumatic patients in the Northern part of the country than in the Southern states. Dr. Mills also observed that acute rheumatic fever is most frequent in stormy areas where air turbulence is common.[3]

The role of humid soil is likewise important. M. Teissier

2. J. M. May, "The Influence of Climate on the Geographical Distribution of Disease," *Medical Biometeorology*, p. 598.
3. C. A. Mills, "Seasonal and Regional Factors in Acute Rheumatic Fever and Rheumatic Disease," *Brit. J. Phys. Med.*, Vol. 10, no. 146 (1936).

and A. Roque noted that French soldiers who had spent long periods of time in wet trenches during World War I often returned as chronic rheumatics.

As a general rule, people living on well-drained permeable terrain where the water does not remain on the surface are less frequently afflicted with rheumatism than persons living on impermeable soil. In a northern country like Great Britain, the impervious clay soils apparently tend to promote rheumatic complaints.

Continental climates with great differences of temperature between summer and winter are disastrous. Laqueur observed that all forms of rheumatic disease are more widespread in Turkey than in other countries, especially in the capital, Ankara, where extremes of temperature prevail. Summers are very hot and winters very cold (down to −5°F). On the other hand, rheumatic disease has a low incidence in equatorial regions, where the heat is constant and the difference between summer and winter is negligible. According to A. Costedoat and J. Jeannest, soldiers in the French Army in North Africa and Indochina suffered less from rheumatic disease than soldiers in France, in spite of the harsher conditions that the soldiers abroad experienced.[4]

On the basis of these various observations, rheumatic patients can be given some climatic advice. One condition is essential: the patient should try to live in a warm, dry, sunny climate with little air turbulence and minimal temperature variations. The climate should not be excessively warm, however, because considerable perspiration followed by evaporation and cooling can be injurious to the patient's health.

4. A. Costedoat and J. Jeannest, *Bull. Soc. Med.*, Vol. 26, no. 1173 (1937).

Geographic Variations in the Incidence of Rickets

Rickets is caused by a vitamin D deficiency. It is a disease occurring in infants and young children, characterized by defective calcification of growing bone, which results in soft, deformed bones. This disease is observed mainly between 40° and 60° latitude. It is very common in Holland, Germany, and Flanders, but rare in Italy. It is absent in the tropics, except among wealthy families who can afford to keep their children out of the sun. It is very common in large industrial cities, where the polluted air prevents the sun's rays from penetrating to the ground below. The incidence of rickets decreases with altitude. It is rare to find rachitic children living in mountainous areas, unless they live on northern slopes that are always shaded. The disease is most common in winter.

In 1921 A. F. Hess and L. J. Unger demonstrated the curative effect of ultraviolet rays on rickets.[5] Ultraviolet rays are necessary for vitamin D formation in the body, and the sun is the greatest source of these rays. Whenever a person lacks exposure to the sun, he runs the risk of becoming rachitic. The geographic distribution of rickets is therefore very closely related to the climatic solar characteristics of a given region. For this reason, England has a higher incidence of rickets than Africa.

Cancer

In an important report published in 1962 by the World Health Organization, a Soviet doctor, A. V. Chaklin, studied

5. A. F. Hess and L. J. Unger: "Interpretation of the Seasonal Variation in Rickets." (*–Am. J. Diseases Children*, 22, 186, 1921).

the causes of cancer in relation to its geographical distribution.[6]

"It is obvious that any serious study of the possible causes of cancer should not disregard the geographic factor in the epidemiology of tumors," wrote Dr. Jack Girond in an analysis of Chaklin's study. But this dread disease can assume countless forms and can be localized almost anywhere in the human body. Do climatic factors play a direct or indirect role in the development of certain cancers? This was the question asked by Doctor Chaklin.

He studied skin cancer first. Several factors can influence or inhibit the appearance of skin cancer. Skin pigmentation, for example, plays an important role. Negroes are less frequently afflicted with this form of cancer than Caucasians. In India, Khanolkar has shown that skin cancer is ten times more frequent among the non-native fair-skinned inhabitants than among the brown-skinned natives.

The type of head protection worn is a factor in the incidence of facial cancer because appropriate head covering provides effective protection against ultraviolet rays. In Central Asia turbans are worn in Tadzhikistan; caps are worn in Uzbekistan; and wide-brimmed fur hats are worn in Turkmenistan. Girond wrote: "It has been established that the incidence of skin cancer is 1.8 times greater in Uzbekistan than in Turkmenistan, yet the average temperature is higher in the latter." The wide-brimmed hats, therefore, provide better protection.

There are some purely climatic factors that act directly on this form of cancer. The frequency of skin cancer increases in tropical countries. According to Dr. Lauraster, this is due to the increased intensity of ultraviolet rays. Climates conducive to cancer of the face are therefore diametrically opposed to climates causing rickets. Ultraviolet rays from the sun help combat rickets, but at the same time favor the

6. Jack Girond, *Semaine Médicale* (January 20, 1963).

development of skin cancer. In fact, ultraviolet rays cause sunburn, which irritates the skin and, if chronic, can actually degenerate into malignant tumors.

This is why skin cancer is more frequent in southern Russia than in northern Russia (30 out of every 100,000 inhabitants in the south, 10 out of every 100,000 in the north). It is rare in Sweden, Denmark, Finland, Norway, and Great Britain, but is common in Bulgaria, Greece, Spain, Italy, the southern part of the United States, and Australia.

We have already discussed the important role of atmospheric pollution in lung cancer. Chaklin confirms our findings: in every country of the world there is more lung cancer among city dwellers than among country dwellers.

Other forms of cancer, and in particular cancer of the digestive system, seem to be related to the eating or chewing habits of various populations. For example, tumors in the mouth are very common in Asian countries where people are in the habit of chewing tobacco or betel leaves. The highest incidence of oral cancer is found in Travancore (India) where 46 percent of cancerous growths are located in the mouth. However, in this part of the world the betel and tobacco "quids" are mixed with chalk, which is very irritating to the mucous membranes.

It is believed that alcoholics are particularly susceptible to cancer of the esophagus. But this form of cancer is also common in cold countries where people tend to drink very hot drinks. Local customs also play their role. About ten years ago in China it was noted that cancer of the esophagus was prevalent in men but that women were spared. The reason is very simple. In that country, the man eats first. The woman must wait until her lord and master has finished. His food is very hot, and hers is almost cold by the time she eats. That is why only the esophagi of males are subject to irritations which can become cancerous.

If cancer of the stomach is less widespread in the tropics than in Europe or North America, there is a higher incidence there of cancer of the liver. Cancer of the liver accounts for 90 percent of the carcinoma among the Bantu as opposed to only 1 percent in France. Nutritional habits are probably not the only reason for this, but they are no doubt a major contributing factor. Chaklin believes that genetic and climatic factors also play a part, but their precise role is not yet known.

Cancer of the breast and cancer of the uterus in women do not seem to be related to climate at first glance. However, it has been noted in Denmark that breast cancer occurs more frequently in cities than in rural districts (32 city cases versus 19 rural cases per 100,000 inhabitants). Although the city climate may be an influential factor, experts feel that local customs such as breast feeding, type of sexual life, etc. are even more important.

Finally, cancer of the thyroid is much more frequent in areas where goiter is a common malady. It is particularly prevalent in mountainous regions such as the Himalayas, the Andes, and the Alps. In this case the climate plays an indirect but definite role.

This very comprehensive study made by the World Health Organization shows that attempts to prevent cancer in the world should take geographical factors into account because they do contribute in the development of certain types of malignant tumors.

"Cancer-Inducing" Houses and Land

"Studies of the distribution of cancer among the population of Le Havre, Loir, and Legangneux have verified a particularly high incidence among the people living on the slopes surrounding the city, where the ground is constantly drenched by streams of running water. The incidence is much lower on the alluvial flat land adjacent to the port, where the water is quickly absorbed by the soil."[7] Does the composition of the subsoil play a role in the origin of cancer? Two recent studies arousing the interest of the medical world proved the topicality of these theories. These studies were made by Dr. William Chen in Hagerstown, Maryland, and Dr. Giacomo Michelangeli in the little village of Buggiano in Italy.

To discover if cancer zones really do exist, Dr. Chen studied every case of cancer occurring in Washington County since the turn of the century. About 100,000 Americans live in this three-hundred-square-mile area. Dr. Chen localized every case and marked it on a map with a red pin. In this way he could see that cancer was not uniformly distributed throughout the county. Cases were grouped in certain areas, certain villages, and even in specific houses. At the turn of the century doctors had created a sort of myth by talking about "cancer-inducing" houses. This premise was not strictly true, because the house itself is not responsible. If it is demolished and a new building constructed on the site, cancer continues to strike in the same place.

Is the subsoil responsible for this? Is it possible that there are harmful radiations emanating from the soil? Chemical analyses of the soil and the subterranean water have been made to see if any radioactivity is present, but this has not yet been confirmed. All we can say is that the zones with the greatest radiation seem to correspond to the areas with the highest incidence of cancer. Dr. Chen's associates believe that "cancer-inducing" houses in Hagerstown county are built on clayey soil and on the banks of streams.

Thirty-five years ago Georges Lakhowsky, a French biophysicist, made a map illustrating cancer in Paris. In his opinion, the frequency of cancer is related to the geology of the terrain. A low incidence of cancer appears in the limestone and sand on the west side of Paris, while a very

7. R. Marot, *Pathologie régionele de la France,* p. 325. (I.N.H., 1958)

high rate shows up in the clay on the southern terrain. Lakhowsky's studies were sharply criticized at the time by Auguste Lumière, who thought that they had been poorly conducted. Nevertheless, it seems that all investigators have found an increased frequency of cancer on terrain situated near waterways or on top of subterranean rivers. We should point out that the interesting research undertaken by Dr. Chen proved only that cancer was unevenly distributed in the areas investigated. Further medical research will be necessary before any valid conclusions can be drawn. Underground radiation is too often cited as a cause of the problem, for lack of better knowledge.

Il paese maledetto

Giacomo Michelangeli, a doctor in a small Italian town, cannot afford to wait. Eighty-five percent of the deaths in his village are caused solely by cancer. Situated in the Abruzzi, a very poor region, the village of Buggiano and its surrounding areas have been called *il paese maledetto*, the cursed land. Cancer here generally involves only the digestive tract: esophagus, stomach, liver. Can the local diet be to blame? The doctor does not believe so. He blames the Buggiano water supply, which is highly radioactive.

However, the Italian Ministry of Health stated that the radioactivity around Buggiano is no greater than in countless other areas of the country. Rome's water, for example, is ten times more radioactive than the water of Buggiano. Professor Seppili, Director of the Perugian Institute of Hygiene, who investigated the matter, concluded that radioactivity was not at fault. In actual fact, the principal cause of Buggiano's misfortune probably lies elsewhere. Heredity may be responsible, because for centuries the inhabitants of Buggiano have intermarried.

It is not impossible for them to have developed a pre-disposition to cancer. All cancer experts are familiar with the important work of Dr. Maud Slye on the predisposition to cancer of certain strains of mice. Occasionally some mice develop cancer spontaneously. Dr. Slye isolated cancerous mice and crossbred them for many generations. Almost all the final descendants of these strains developed cancer spontaneously.

Studies by three American doctors, A. S. Warthin, J. J. Hauser, and C. V. Weller, on the genealogy of the G. family, which had all too often suffered malignant tumors, revealed similar tendencies. When the genealogical tree of the G. family was complete, doctors observed that of 174 members who lived to be adults, 41 had developed cancer. This means that 24 percent of the members of one family suffered from cancer.

The case is obviously exceptional and extreme, but so is the situation in Buggiano. It is possible that special soil and water conditions in this small Italian town joined forces with some hereditary factors to cause this affliction. Only the future and further research will be able to settle this question.

Lack of Magnesium?

In 1930 Dr. Robinet thought he had formally proved the correlation existing in Alsace-Lorraine between the amount of magnesium in the soil and the development of cancer in the population there. To the east of the Vosges Mountains there is very little magnesium in the soil and a high cancer mortality rate. To the west of the Vosges the soil is rich in magnesium, and there is a relatively low mortality rate.

Professor Pierre Delbet and his colleagues later repeated

8. John H. Woodburn, *Cancer, the Search for its Origins* (New York: Holt, Rinehart and Winston, 1964), p. 53.

this opinion. On March 13, 1951, Professor Delbet made this alarming statement to the members of the Academy of Medicine: "The real cause of the increase in cancer is that the soil is lacking in magnesium. Every year the harvests remove considerable amounts of this metal. It has been estimated that 49 pounds per acre are absorbed by a good sugar-beet crop. . . . Magnesium is particularly important, because it is one of the trace elements in tissue."

Delbet and his colleagues provided the Academy with very convincing proof. Their geological maps and graphs of cancer mortality corresponded almost exactly: hence the conclusion that where the soil is poor in magnesium, cancer is common. Similarly in 1941 and 1942, Depeyre, a colleague of Delbet's, showed that in 12 regions with soil rich in magnesium, 66 deaths out of 1,000 were caused by cancer. On the other hand, in 12 regions with almost no magnesium in the soil, the number of deaths from cancer spiraled to 101 in every 1,000 deaths. In Delbert's opinion, the solution is simple: increase the amount of magnesium in food where it is inadequate and above all, add supplementary amounts of this valuable but disappearing metal to fertilizer. "I am absolutely sure," he concluded, "that by maintaining adequate magnesium deposits in the soil, we will be able to diminish greatly the incidence of cancer in a few years." [9]

This opinion is no doubt worthy of consideration. However, it has never been unanimously accepted. Those experts who have regarded it with skepticism have sound reasons to support their incredulity. The Parisian basin and those areas to the east that are the most affected by cancer are the areas where the largest cities are located. And large cities are known to generate carcinogenic pollution. Furthermore, those areas also have the greatest tobacco consumption. This in itself can account for their high rate of cancer of the respira-

9. Pierre Delbet, et al., "Appauvrissement du sol en magnésium et ses conséquences," *Bulletin de l'Académie de Médicine* (March 13, 1951).

tory tract. Finally, the demographic experts whom I consulted believe that any statistics linking cancer to a lack of magnesium are ignoring natural mortality factors. "What is cancer, anyway?" they ask. It is a disease primarily of the elderly. Moreover, they add, a map of France showing the distribution of age will correspond almost exactly with a map showing the distribution of mortality from cancer. The "young" areas have fewer deaths from cancer than the "old" ones.

Goiter

The relationship between soil and disease is an extremely complex problem. The influences of the soil, the weather, water, population density, and standard of living are closely interwoven. Cancer is not the only disease resulting from a combination of all these factors.

Dr. Marot's study of goiter is very informative. We know that goiter is a benign tumor of the thyroid gland characterized by hypertrophy of this gland. This disease has a very irregular geographic distribution. For example, Dr. M. Rhein outlined two very distinct regions in France where goiter is common. One lies along the banks of the Rhine and its tributary the Ill, the other in the foothills and valleys of the Vosges. Separating these two regions is an unaffected area.[10] There, wrote Marot, the well water is excellent, the land is fertile, and the inhabitants live in comfortable, hygienic conditions. However, along the banks of the Rhine and the Ill, where goiter is endemic, the porous, permeable subsoil is unable to prevent the water from becoming contaminated. Several years ago Dr. Freyss studied the school

10. M. Rhein: "La répartition géographique du goitre en Alsace" (The Geographical Distribution of Goiter in Alsace—*Soc. Méd. du Bas-Rhin,* meeting of April 13, 1935).

children of Strasbourg. He discovered two facts: first, that the children with goiters were drinking polluted well water while the non-goitrous children were drinking water from the city supply, which was under the control of the local Health Department; and second, that the children with goiters harbored many intestinal parasites which seemed to have a definite hypertrophic effect on the thyroid gland.

Marot concluded his study with these generalizations: "The areas in France where goiter is endemic are extensions of the large endemic zones covering southern and western Germany. . . . continuing into Switzerland and extending as far as Czechoslovakia. . . . This is a typical example of "border pathology," *i.e.*, an area open to all invasions, whether military or morbid, coming from the east or the north."[11]

Marot does not go into the matter of diet as a cause of goiter, but the World Health Organization in 1960 published a study which reported that all the evidence points to a lack of iodine in food and drinking water as the primary cause of simple endemic goiter.

The goiter areas of the United States are primarily along the whole Appalachian Mountain range, in the states bordering the Great Lakes, and the western states of Montana, Idaho, Oregon, and Washington. This exemplifies the fact, as F. C. Kelly and W. W. Snedden point out in their study of the geographical distribution of goiter, that proximity to the sea does not necessarily guarantee freedom from the disease. An interesting explanation for this is offered by students of iodine chemistry who have found that areas where goiter is prevalent, whether at high or low altitude, are those which have been subjected to intense flooding or glaciation and from which the soil iodine has been washed out and has not yet been sufficiently replaced by airborne oceanic iodine. An examination of the very high-rate goiter areas in the United States and Europe shows a close correlation between those areas and regions that were heavily glaciated.

11. Marot, *op. cit.*, p. 236.

Although in recent times goiter has been largely overcome through the increasing use of iodized salt, the disease is still recognized as a serious regional health problem.

The Soil's Electrical Field

The soil's texture can either propagate disease or protect its inhabitants. The electrical fields created in the earth's crust play an important role in these influences. In Piéry's classical *Traité de Climatologie biologique et medicale* Y. Pech writes: "Experience shows that creatures living in contact with the soil are in the same electrical state as this soil." [12] Variations in the earth's electric fields seem to influence our health. The electric field is negative near waterfalls, river rapids, in caves, holes in the ground, and where water oozes down walls. Elsewhere it is positive.

Pech has shown that this field has a considerable effect on animals. Sheep and ewes, for example, only appear content when on land that is in an electrically positive field. Here they are always gamboling and frolicking. But if the land is in an electrically negative field, they stop their play, lie down and appear anxious. The mystery of such different behavior has not been solved. Pech concluded his study by saying: "The slightest variation in the soil's electrical state can cause major disorders in living creatures."

The influence of soil on man's health remains a mystery. It is a highly complex problem, for the soil of a given region has not only a specific physico-chemical composition, but also a specific electrical potential, radioactivity, and magnetic field. Today we are just beginning to explore the possible influence of these factors on men and animals.

---

12. Y. Pech, *Physioclimatologie générale des climats*, p. 630.

Extremes of Climate

Man is a curious, adventuresome creature. He wants to go everywhere. Climbing the highest mountains, crossing barren deserts, exploring the poles, and now landing on the moon are dreams that he has brought to reality. But today courage and the desire to test endurance are no longer the only motivations of those who want to conquer nature's best-defended outposts Once today's explorers reach a destination, they remain and settle there. Some pursue military objectives, others are interested in commercial enterprises. Man's journeys into the most extreme climates force him to adapt to these climates in order to survive during prolonged stays.

A new branch of medicine has developed to answer these needs. Studies on acclimatization during the past few years have been very informative about man's ability to adapt to three different kinds of extreme climate: high altitude, severe cold, and intense heat. Dr. Rivolier, who has been a member of numerous scientific expeditions in the Himalayas and to Adélie Coast (Antarctica), published some extremely pertinent observations on this subject.

Mountain Sickness

As one climbs above sea level, atmospheric pressure, temperature, and water vapor all decrease. The winds become stronger, and the amount of solar radiation is intensified. Up to an altitude of 6,500 feet solar radiation increases by 2 to 4 percent every 300 feet. Over 6,500 feet it increases an additional 1 percent every 300 feet. At this altitude the intensity of the sun's reflected rays can cause cutaneous and ocular burns if special precautions are not taken. Ocular burns are more frequent on snow and ice.

At very high altitudes the cosmic rays must be taken into consideration, although their influence on human physiology is still not precisely known.

The most important factor in high-altitude climates is the gradual decrease in oxygen caused by rarefaction of the atmosphere. This decreased oxygen level is one of the principal causes of high-altitude sickness (known as mountain sickness). The altitude at which this disease starts to affect the organism varies with each individual. But over an altitude of approximately 16,000 feet everyone feels the effect. The symptoms are as follows:

"The subject feels a desire to breathe deeply but has the sensation of being unable to do so. He experiences respiratory difficulties with the slightest effort. Other symptoms include drowsiness, asthenia, headache, and vertigo.

Very often the subject complains of feeling cold and has digestive disorders. He is pale or cyanosed. His pulse is rapid and slightly irregular; his blood pressure can rise or fall abruptly. In rare cases death may ensue if the subject remains at high altitude and is unable to adapt." [13]

Acclimatization to High Altitudes

Even trained athletes find it very difficult to perform well at altitudes higher than 6,000 to 10,000 feet above sea level. The Olympic Games were held in 1968 in Mexico City, which is 10,000 feet above sea level. All the competitors had good reason to be apprehensive. As early as 1965 some athletes were sent to test the tracks. Their performances, especially in long-distance events, were very

13. J. Rivolier, "Physiopathologie de l'altitude," *Encyclopédie médico-chirurgicale*, Volume: *Agents physiques*.

poor. A great champion like Ron Clark took one minute longer than his regular time to run 5,000 meters and finished the race exhausted. The organizers were worried that no athletes would even be able to complete the marathon.

There was only one solution: acclimatization. Man has hidden resources which, given time, permit him to adapt to the harshest conditions. Radical changes can occur in his body, enabling him to establish a new physiological equilibrium.

The head physician of France's National Institute of Sport, Dr. Jean Andrivet, undertook a very revealing experiment. Some of the athletes who had been selected for the pre-Olympic trials in Mexico were sent first to train at Font-Rameu, a health resort situated in the Pyrenees at an altitude of 7,000 feet. For several days they ran, jumped, and threw weights. When they arrived in Mexico, they were able to perform up to standard. Their bodies had had time to adapt to the high altitude. Another group of French athletes who had not spent a training period at Font-Rameu participated in the trials soon after disembarking from their plane. Their performances were much poorer than their regular performances at low altitude. They suffered from shortness of breath and had no competitive spirit.

The doctors in charge of the health and welfare of the French athletes learned a valuable lesson from this experiment. They realized the necessity of letting the athletes train at a high altitude for the coming Olympics. So in 1968 Font-Rameu became the center for French athletics.

Man's ability to adapt to high altitudes has long been proven by the populations of the Andes and the Himalayas, who live at altitudes of 13,000 to 16,000 feet without any apparent difficulty. But can a man who has always lived at sea level adapt to life at this altitude? Yes, provided that he acclimatizes himself gradually. "A subject used to living at sea level who suddenly finds himself at an altitude of 20,000 to 23,000 feet (by using a decompression chamber, for example) will faint and show other serious symptoms that can lead to death if he is not given supplementary amounts of oxygen. On the other hand, a climber who has been training for several weeks at gradually higher altitudes will be able to live almost normally if placed in similar conditions." [14]

It takes approximately ten days to acclimatize to an altitude of 10,000 feet, and five to six weeks to acclimatize to an altitude of 20,000 feet. Acclimatization is rarely possible over 23,000 feet. There are some individuals, hypersensitive to high altitudes, who never adapt

"Cursed Places"

The problem of acclimatization at high altitudes contains some puzzling elements. For example, it is not always permanent. Loss of tolerance to the altitude may occur, suddenly, causing a condition known as "chronic mountain sickness." This is a strange malady, occurring not only in foreigners who have been living at the altitude for a long time but also in the natives. For example, on the Andes plateau, it is not uncommon for a native to find that he is suddenly unable to live at his accustomed altitude. This generally occurs after the age of forty. The man suddenly loses the altitude tolerance that was believed to be an integral part of his organism, his legacy from generations and generations of mountain-dwelling relatives. If he does not leave his plateau, he will die.

Even stranger events can occur, leading investigators to question whether scarcity of oxygen is the only cause of mountain sickness. For generations mountain people have believed that in the hollows of mountains are "cursed places" that cause those who venture into them to become ill.

14. *Ibid.*

These are not mere legends; they have been confirmed several times. In the Andean Belt these places are called *lugares de puma*. What happens in one of them seems magical. A native who until then has felt well suddenly loses his breath and feels as though he is going to die. But— and herein lies the mystery—if he overcomes his indisposition and climbs above the spot, his malaise disappears. Yet at higher altitudes the oxygen concentration is lower! Lack of oxygen therefore does not adequately explain these "cursed places."

Mont Blanc in France also has its "cursed place," yet I do not know of any such spots in the Himalayas, the world's highest mountains.

What causes the deadly effect in these places? Perhaps certain electrical phenomena in the atmosphere (especially atmospheric ionization) present anomalies that provoke disorders in addition to those caused by the lack of oxygen.

Adaptation to Cold Climates

Man's body is poorly equipped to tolerate the cold. In the hypothalamus we have two thermoregulatory centers: one reacts to cold, the other to heat. But they have very limited powers and do not provide adequate protection against extreme temperatures. Animals have fur or plumage that conserves body heat, but our bodies have recourse to only one adaptative reaction. Circulation can be modified by *vasoconstriction:* the surface capillaries constrict, which reduces the blood supply to the skin and limits the loss of heat. This defense mechanism enables man to perform tasks with his hands exposed in freezing weather, provided that the rest of his body is well protected. But vasoconstriction only works on the surface of the body. If the cold is too intense, man runs the risk of frostbite, which can afflict him before any real pain sets in. The frozen area becomes white and insensitive, and the subject has the impression of no longer being able to feel it. It is not until he tries to rewarm the area that severe pain is felt. Generally even after healing, frostbite leaves the area sensitive to cold.

The whole body can only tolerate sudden exposure to intense cold for a very short time. Witness the grim proof in the Nazi extermination camps. With very rare exceptions prisoners exposed naked for several hours at below-zero temperatures died very quickly.

But it is not necessary to recall the horrors of these death camps to discuss the effects of freezing on man. An explorer lost in an Antarctic blizzard or a mountaineer who has fallen into a crevasse suffers the same fate. "The subject shivers intensely and has violent muscular pains mainly in the area of the neck. As his deep body temperature decreases, he experiences muscular rigidity, and seizures of an epileptic nature occur. His respiration and pulse become irregular. He eventually falls into a coma, and death ensues." [15]

If the subject is rescued in time, the only effective treatment is rapid but gentle rewarming by immersing him in a warm bath with the water at about 110°F. Frostbitten areas should be warmed in the same way. Massaging should be avoided at all costs because it increases pain and edema and is of no benefit.

Adaptation to Heat

Our nervous system adapts better to heat. When the body is very warm, the blood capillaries of the skin dilate and allow more heat to escape. This process is called vasodilatation. The subject also perspires; and as the perspiration evaporates, it lowers the body temperature. Conse-

15. *Ibid.,* "Les Accidents dus au Froid."

quently, the whole body works to combat the heat. This can be verified by measuring the amount of salt and water lost by perspiration; when the body is exposed to heat over a period of time these amounts are greatly increased.

However, as with exposure to cold, the human organism rapidly reaches its limits of toleration. Prolonged exposure to excessively high temperature can cause heat prostration. Ordinary heat prostration is characterized by high fever, cramps, shortness of breath, and palpitation. If exposure to heat continues, the disorder becomes much more serious. The subject becomes very pale. His temperature rises to 105°F or higher, and he becomes severely dehydrated. Profound shock and heart failure may follow. Several years ago in the Sahara desert, some foolhardy young soldiers ventured off in a truck that subsequently broke down. After an hour's wait in the scorching sun, some of them, terrified by the heat, left the protective shelter of their machine and set out on foot across the sand. They died of heat prostration about a half-mile from their truck. Those who had been wise enough to stay in the shade were rescued.

Man appears to be the creature most unable to tolerate extremes of temperature. But fortunately, his brain is an unsurpassed thermoregulator and can devise thousands of ways to protect him from extremes of temperature. He builds shelters, makes protective clothing, and has learned how to create artificial methods of heating and cooling the air.

For man, housing and clothing are a climatic necessity, so imperative that for many years it seemed too obvious to be studied by scientists. But today this is no longer the case. Housing and clothing have been incorporated into the domain of science, as we shall see later.

The Micro-Climate of Cities

By creating enormous, sprawling cities, man has gradually modified the climate in which he lives. A large urban center has different atmospheric conditions from the areas surrounding it. This is so self-evident that meteorological stations are always constructed on the outskirts of cities.

As a general rule, the temperature in a large city is two or three degrees higher than in the surrounding countryside. The climate is not as severe in winter because of the heat generated by homes and factories. The buildings conserve this heat, and provide protection against winds.

In summer cities present an altogether different picture. The heat accumulated during the day by the walls of buildings and the asphalt on pavements is released in the evening. Every Parisian, Roman, and New Yorker has experienced the stifling, oppressive August evenings of his city. In humid weather this heat soon becomes unbearable.

We tend to think that one climate extends over large areas. But local characteristics within a region create their own small climates, which meteorologists term "micro-climates." A city is a micro-climate with characteristic atmospheric and meteorological conditions. Summer showers over major large cities are a good example of this. These showers fall only over cities because the cities are responsible for their formation. All day long, in summer, the heat from buildings and roads creates strong convection currents, which attract the more humid air from the surrounding countryside. The water vapor rises, becomes cool, and in the evening falls on the sweltering city as a refreshing shower.

Even within a city there are distinct climatic variations. The center of a town, for example, warms and cools more slowly than the periphery. Every neighborhood has its own special micro-climate. A study made by the Research Council of St. Thomas' Hospital in London indicates that rheumatic patients almost always live less than a mile from the Thames river. Similarly, in New York State there are more cases of rheumatic disease in areas close to the sea, where the microclimate has a high humidity.

London Mailmen

Some very common maladies can differ from city to city and even according to the neighborhood, street, or floor on which we live.

A comprehensive study of bronchitis illustrates this point well. This disease is characterized by an inflammation of the bronchi caused by infection or pollutants in the air. The bronchi become blocked by mucus that has not been properly drained by the tracheal cilia. Acute bronchitis is characterized by fever, chest pain, choking sensations, and painful, interminable coughing fits. Many heavy smokers and elderly people suffer from chronic bronchitis. This disease is much more prevalent in cities than in the country.

In 1954 studies by J. Pemberton and C. Goldberg indicated that among males from 45 to 65 years of age the death rate from bronchitis was 61 per 100,000 inhabitants living in rural districts. But this figure rose to 114 deaths per 100,-000 in cities. Polluted air is considered to be the harmful contributing factor.[16]

Some interesting statistics concerning London mailmen were compiled by D. D. Reid and A. S. Fairbairn. They studied the medical records of 565 mailmen who had been forced to retire prematurely because of chronic bronchitis contracted while working. However, the number of mailmen afflicted varied according to the districts in which they had

16. J. Pemberton and C. Goldberg, "Air Pollution and Bronchitis," *Brit. Med. J.*, Vol. 2, no. 567 (1954).

their delivery routes. The rate rose steadily from the south-west of London, where it was lowest, to the northeast, where it was highest.

Apparently the Postal Administration did try to have all their employees work under identical conditions. The temperature and humidity were more or less the same in every district. But they had forgotten to consider the smoke.

The prevailing wind in London blows from the west-southwest, and consequently carries all the smoke in the direction of the northeast section of the city. The number of mailmen suffering from bronchitis in a given area corresponded to the level of the area's air pollution. A similar phenomenon was observed in relation to the frequency of lung cancer in London.

A 12-year survey, ending in 1960, of deaths in and around Nashville, Tennessee, showed the relation between air pollution levels and deaths from respiratory disease: more deaths from breathing ailments occurred in those sections of the city which were subjected to the heaviest air pollution.

Where we live is therefore very important for our health. Dr. Reid reached the following conclusion: "In a group of men doing the same job for the same pay under the same conditions of service, disabling respiratory disease is directly related to the micro-climate in which these men work." [17] The observations by Reid and Fairbairn underline the importance of town planning for public health.

Emphysema is the *fastest growing case of death* in the United States. There has been a 17-fold increase between 1950 and 1966. As with respiratory disease in general, the urban death rate is about twice as high as the rural one, reflecting the connection between emphysema and air pollution.

A study of autopsies on 300 residents of heavily polluted St. Louis, Missouri, and 300 residents of relatively pollution-free Winnipeg, Canada, showed that, even when smoking

17. D. D. Reid and A. S. Fairbairn, "The Natural History of Chronic Bronchitis," *Lancet*, no. 1147 (May 1958).

histories were taken into consideration, emphysema was more prevalent in St. Louis than Winnipeg; it developed earlier and progressed more rapidly.

The Micro-Climate of Buildings

One English climatologist, J. K. Page, made this wise comment: "The majority of people in the world spend at least half their lives in the artificial climates that exist within the walls of buildings." [18] Man's health is determined therefore just as much by the indoor climate of his home and workplace as it is by the outdoor climate. Hence we should know how to create the healthiest climate around ourselves.

The construction of dwellings poses many climatological problems, the first being the materials used. Arsène d'Arsonval, a French biologist, observed that the construction of modern concrete apartment buildings has created a new predicament because concrete does not allow the atmosphere's electrical waves to penetrate. The buildings thus become Faraday cages. Not enough time has elapsed for us to determine what the effects of this type of construction may be on the human organism.

Shortly before the war, Lakhowsky, a biophysicist, stated his belief that there existed "cancer-inducing houses," as we have seen. But in his opinion construction materials were not the cause. He believed that the danger lay in certain harmful rays coming from the soil.

The total environment created by the four annual seasons should be considered when deciding which construction materials and methods to use. The choice is difficult because the ideal materials for summer are unsuitable for winter, and vice versa. For economic reasons there is now a tendency to

18. J. K. Page, "An Introduction to Urban Biometeorology," *Medical Biometeorology* (1963), p. 655.

construct buildings with thin walls. This means that in winter a great deal of heat is lost, and in summer the residents swelter because the walls provide poor insulation from the outside heat. Old houses are often very pleasant in this respect. In both winter and summer their thick walls act as an insulating element between the outside and the inside.

Asthma and Old Dwellings

Nevertheless, old houses have their shortcomings. For example, the humid wood of old residences often causes allergies. H. Varekamp has been conducting a very enlightening study on this question since 1958 in Leiden. Part of the Netherlands, as we know, is situated below or right at sea level; therefore humidity poses a great problem for construction. In 70 percent of the houses built before 1918 the wood used has rotted—especially the wooden floors of these houses. Varekamp discovered a very significant relationship between asthma and houses with old wood floors. All allergy specialists know that some people cannot inhale dust without immediately beginning to choke, and the dust created by old wood has very intense allergenic qualities. Tests have been made by injecting samples of this dust into the patients' skin. The surface of the skin immediately turned a bright red color, proof of an allergic reaction.[19]

Recently Dr. Voorhorst and his team found another cause of asthmatic attacks—the mites that often infest old floors. After countless tests it was discovered that a certain type of mite, the *Dermatophagoides scheremetevski*, secretes a toxic product which, when combined with dust, affects asthmatic sufferers.

In Amsterdam, The Hague, and Rotterdam, people suf-

19. H. Varekamp, "De betekenis van houtrot voor de behuizing," *Tijdschr. Soc. Geneesk.* (1958), p. 649.

fering asthmatic attacks often have to move from their old
residences and relocate in new apartments in order to be free
of their complaints. The conclusions reached by Dutch
doctors can obviously be applied to the old houses of other
countries.

The Best Direction for Buildings to Face

One important point remains to be mentioned: the best
orientation for buildings. The first factor to be considered is
the sun. In northern cities of the Northern Hemisphere, the
best orientation would be southeast. In winter, when the sun
is low on the horizon, its rays can easily penetrate into rooms
and warm them. In summer the sun is too high in the sky
to penetrate an apartment facing southeast. Therefore apartments with this orientation are not as hot as those facing
southwest, which become suffocating from the late afternoon
sun. Apartments facing north are generally the most unfavorable because, with so little sunlight entering them, they tend
to become damp.

It goes without saying that the amount of heat and sunlight we should have in our homes depends primarily on the
climate in which we live. In the Scandinavian countries the
windows should be large to take maximum advantage of the
light. In southern countries small windows are more suitable
because they prevent excessive sun from entering in summer.

As a general rule, the correlation between lack of sunshine and rickets and the claims made for ultraviolet therapy
in curing tuberculosis indicate that our homes should be
exposed to as much sunlight as possible. However, it should
be noted that virtually no ultraviolet light penetrates normal
windowpanes. The physiological benefits consist mainly of
the "euphoria" derived from being in a pleasant, sunny
environment.

Equivalent Environments

The sense of well-being, feeling neither too hot nor too cold, breathing air which is not too humid nor too dry, differs with each person's temperament. Meteorologists term this feeling "comfort," and they have tried to transform the subjective notion of it into a scientific definition. "We have tried to determine the 'comfort' characteristics of an environment. This is rather difficult because feelings of warmth and cold depend on a great number of factors: temperature, humidity, and air movement, as well as clothing, muscular activity, nutrition, age, general body build, degree of acclimatization, respiratory rate, the temperature of the surrounding walls, etc. This data, however, does have an important practical application in the air conditioning of rooms. In the United States different atmospheric characteristics giving the same objective sensation have been called 'equivalent environments.'" [20]

Accidents Due to Temperature

We have often heard people say, "The cold paralyzes me" or, "The heat exhausts me." These sayings reflect more than a subjective reaction; some very serious physiological consequences can ensue from stress caused by heat or cold. Two investigators, H. Vernon and T. Bedford, studied the daily number of accidents occurring in a large munitions factory during World War I. It appeared that heat over 75°F caused a 23 percent increase in accidents. Cold below 50°F was even more disastrous. The accident rate then rose 35 percent above average. The same investigators observed that most

20. Rivolier, *op. cit.*, p. 57.

underground mining accidents occurred at either the warmest places in the mine or in areas exposed to currents of freezing air. The accident rate under these circumstances rose alarmingly and was 61 to 72 percent higher than the average accident rate.[21]

Other biological tests enable us to study how each of us reacts to the stress of heat or cold. One test evaluating biological reactions to cold seems like a game, but it is not. It is called the finger test, and it allows us to judge the effectiveness of our thermoregulatory powers. The test is as follows: when a healthy person immerses a finger in iced water, the skin temperature of this finger rapidly falls to 32°F. But fifteen minutes later the skin temperature spontaneously rises again to 41–42°F. With continued immersion the finger temperature fluctuates slowly between 32°F and 41–42°F. The reason for these oscillations is not known, but they indicate good functioning of the internal thermoregulatory powers that enable the organism to defend itself successfully against the cold.

Sometimes the temperature of the immersed finger remains at 32°F. A sort of red patch then forms on the finger. In this case the subject is probably hypersensitive to the cold. He should be extremely careful if he exposes his body to cold, and should avoid swimming in icy water at all costs.

The amount of humidity in the air is almost as important as the temperature. Air that is too dry dehydrates the mucosa of the nose and throat, and the subject is more easily irritated by surrounding dust. But a hot, moist atmosphere is even more unbearable. N. H. Mackworth, a British physician, showed that too much humidity in the air interferes with intellectual effort, especially concentration. Eleven competent radio operators who usually made very few errors were observed in a hot, humid atmosphere. They began making more

21. H. Vernon and T. Bedford, "The Relation of Atmospheric Conditions to the Working Capacity and the Accident Rate of Miners," *Rept. Ind. Fatigue Research Board*, no. 39 (1927).

mistakes. As the heat and humidity increased, they made more and more errors. They were making an average of 12 errors per hour at 85°F. This figure increased to 95 errors per hour at 105°F.[22]

In a good building it is normal to maintain an average humidity of 50 percent. But all too often this humidity increases as a result of household activities (cooking, bathing, showering, etc.). To prevent humidity from disturbing our feeling of well-being and staining the walls as it condenses, effective ventilation is necessary.

Comfort and Health

Comfort and health are not synonymous. This may seem paradoxical, but it is nevertheless true. Without realizing it, man occasionally assures his comfort at the expense of his health.

This is a universal trait. In Nigeria doctors were upset about the severe epidemics of meningitis which used to appear in winter. What was the main cause of these epidemics? In winter the natives huddled together at night in the same hut to avoid the cold. The spread of germs from one individual to another was very prevalent. It was extremely difficult to convince the Nigerians to live in separate huts in winter as they did in summer because the cold winter weather made their separate dwellings less attractive than the communal household.

The conflict between comfort and health occurs in our modern residences. If we shut ourselves in during the winter, we reduce the stress from the cold and at the same time we increase the heat indoors. But we run the risk of substituting other dangerous elements for the cold. The amount of bac-

22. N. H. Mackworth, "Effects of Heat on Wireless Operators," *Brit. J. Ind. Med.*, Vol. 3, no. 143 (1946).

teria in the rooms increases; tobacco smoke accumulates, irritating the throat and bronchi; the humidity rises and makes the atmosphere oppressive; and if there is not enough humidity, the dry air irritates the mucosa of the respiratory tract. This is why it is not recommended to cut off all fresh air during the cold season.

The Best Heating Methods

A major problem is to have properly heated buildings without endangering our health. How can artificial sources of heat best be used to combat cold? Heating engineers offer some solutions.

Some factors causing loss of heat are hard to control. For instance, if we live in a building with very thin walls, more heat will be lost than from well-insulated buildings with solid walls. If the building is old and the doors and windows are improperly sealed when closed, drafts will cause a great loss of heat. But this is not difficult to correct. Walls that are too thin can be reinforced with layers of fiber glass, which provide good insulation against both cold and noise.

Here are some fundamental guidelines to assure better efficiency from the type of heating equipment installed. As we know, warm air tends to rise and cold air to descend. Cold air enters primarily through lower openings in dwellings, mainly through the windows. It is therefore recommended, where possible, to place the source of heat under a window. In this way the cold air is warmed as it enters the room. It then rises and creates a flow of pleasant air.

Practical advice concerning different methods of heating can be deduced from this single law. Hot-air heating systems are rarely effective unless the air vent is placed as low as possible in the room. If the discharge outlet is placed high in the room, the floor remains cold and the ceiling becomes very warm. Consequently, our feet freeze while our heads become congested. To avoid this situation, there is a tendency now to place the heating system beneath or within the floor. Floor heating either by electricity or by embedded hot water pipes has proved to be very effective. However, care should be taken to ensure that the temperature of the floor does not exceed 80°F, for temperatures greater than this can occasionally cause problems. People whose work requires them to spend long hours on their feet—nurses working in hospitals, for example, which are heated by this method—often complain of swollen ankles and legs

Air Conditioning

The ideal solution for obtaining a comfortable indoor temperature is to supply the rooms with a constant flow of air during all seasons. This is air conditioning. The term is used today mainly to designate procedures that lower the temperature, but it can also act as a warming element. True air conditioning, however, should imply full control of all indoor atmospheric conditions that affect our well-being and health: temperature of the air, its moisture content, pollution level, etc.

As it is used today, air conditioning does have certain disadvantages besides its cost of installation. Once installed throughout a whole building, closed-circuit air conditioning not only recirculates the conditioned air from one room to another, but it also recirculates the accumulated bacteria and smoke, etc. This becomes a serious problem in hospitals. Some users complain occasionally of the unpleasant noise that air conditioning makes as it passes from room to room. J. K. Page, a British hygiene engineer, mentions these disadvantages but adds that they can be overcome. For example, air conditioning should not recirculate the same air continuously in a closed circuit. The air should be renewed regularly by bringing in outside air so gradually that the inside temperature is not affected. "The ideal solution is for the air-conditioning unit to take in a fresh air supply equivalent to one-fifth of the total amount of air circulating at every circuit," says Page.

Will we ever be able to control *all* the atmospheric conditions within our dwellings? In the opinion of Dr. de Rudder, this is neither possible nor desirable. Some very subtle effects of the weather are felt in rooms with hermetically sealed doors and windows. Even in bed (the smallest and most stable micro-climate) a patient with rheumatism, arthritis, or an amputated limb can feel changes of weather. It is difficult for us to control electrical impulses in the air or the exchanges between ions, those particles that have lately been discovered to be so important for our health. The effects of cosmic conditions can scarcely be controlled either, as we shall see in the next chapter. This is normal: an organism living completely isolated from outside influences dies. Proof of this was demonstrated in a famous experiment, the Simplon tunnel: animals sheltered from all external changes by the great protection afforded by that mountain soon died. The electrical exchanges had become too inadequate for them to survive.

Astronauts' Living Quarters

There is one micro-climate that creates an entirely new set of environmental problems—that of space vehicles. Tromp devoted a whole chapter of his book *Medical Biometeorology* to a discussion of this topic. One specialist, Donald R. Ekberg, described to what extent the astronaut's environment is altered when he sets out in space. Atmospheric pressure, temperature, air constituents are all radically changed. The hermetically sealed space cabin obviously manages to maintain these vital atmospheric factors in a constant state. But the effects of the lack of gravity that is experienced once the astronauts are several miles from the earth's surface have not been mastered. Space physicians are worried lest *all* the harmful rays from the cosmos penetrate the sealed walls of space capsules. There are still many unanswered questions in space exploration.

F. A. Brown and his colleagues in America have emphasized the biological role of the magnetic fields' effects. How will man's body react when placed for a long time under abnormal gravitational and magnetic conditions? This is only one of the questions that interplanetary voyages will answer.

Climatic Role of Clothing

Clothing is man's oldest, most permanent, and closest form of protection against bad weather. It is of major importance from a climatic point of view. For several years researchers have been trying to establish scientific norms in this ancient field previously dominated by fancy. Consideration of the clothing worn by both primitive and civilized populations suggests that protection from atmospheric conditions was not the only factor responsible for its development. Even more important than climatic usefulness were the influences of fashion, social tradition, and religious customs.[23]

Today scientists are studying the influence of various types of clothing on our health. In this way certain recognized effects can be explained and inaccurate beliefs can be rectified. Here are some examples taken from the works of E. T. Renbourn, who has spent a considerable amount of time studying this question.

23. E. T. Renbourn, "Influence of Different Types of Clothing," *Medical Biometeorology* (1963), p. 434.

Do we know what makes a garment warm? Until recently most of the fabrics used for our clothing were derived either from animal materials, such as wool, or from vegetable fibers, such as cotton and linen. Nowadays a large variety of clothing materials are made from synthetic fibers. These synthetic fabrics accumulate a high content of static electricity. We have all seen sparks flying from a nylon garment when it is taken off in the dark. Some people maintain that these static charges are of physiological value in relieving rheumatism. According to Dr. Renbourn, "This assumption has no great scientific foundation." In reality, the warmth of a cloth is not due to the physical properties of its fibers but primarily to the amount of air that becomes enmeshed and imprisoned in the interstices between the fibers. This trapped air is warmed by our bodies and provides insulation from the outside temperature. Hence we have the impression that the garment is "warm."

Wool, for example, when viewed microscopically, is composed of tiny, overlapping elastic scales. This enables it to enmesh and retain air, making it superior to most other fibers. It has the best "aerodynamic drag" because its fibers tend to prevent air from moving within or passing through it. In sheep's wool nature has provided a wonderful weapon against the vagaries of atmospheric temperature.

Garments are also designed to provide the body with maximum insulation from humidity. In rain, wool and cotton fabrics absorb large amounts of water in the interstices between their fibers. It is possible for a thick woolen coat to double its weight without any dampness reaching the skin. Synthetic fabrics absorb much less water and therefore give the wearer an unpleasantly damp feeling very quickly.

The ideal fabric for excessively damp weather contains fibers that have been treated with silicones or fatty acids. This treatment changes the surface tension of the fibers in such a way that the water forms drops on top of the garment instead of seeping into the fabric.

Strict scientific tests on the color of garments have shown that this is not as important as was formerly believed for our well-being and comfort. White reflects the sun's infrared rays better than black. But white clothing has more or less the same effect as black because the fabric's surface is not smooth enough to act as a reflector.

The Search for an Ideal Fabric

Some investigators believe that a fiber coated with metal retains body heat best because it reflects heat back to the body. For several years manufacturers have been testing fabrics "metallized" with aluminum as linings in raincoats or as lightweight winter suits. But these clothes have not become popular. It is acknowledged, however, that a blanket with a metallized film does maintain a higher skin temperature than a regular blanket. But these fabrics have the disadvantage of being impermeable to water vapor from perspiration.

De Rudder noted that "there are some garments containing metallic threads to protect the body from electromagnetic waves. These garments become a sort of 'walking Faraday cage.' " [24] But is it beneficial or harmful to prevent these rays from reaching our bodies? This question has not yet been answered.

Technicians are trying in every possible way to develop the ideal fabric for the most functional garment. It is possible that this ideal garment may be very far removed in both fabric and style from what we now wear.

Some scientists feel that the garment will be made entirely of inexpensive synthetic materials so that it can be discarded after one wearing. The fabric would then be dissolved in solvents and reutilized. Other investigators claim that research on the ideal garment is all in vain because the

24. B. de Rudder, *op. cit.*, p. 263.

future of clothing actually lies in its gradual disappearance. In their opinion, clothing is a hindrance in summer and will become purposeless in winter as man lives more and more in a controlled environment. This opinion seems highly exaggerated, to say the least. Even if nudity is accepted on hygienic, esthetic, and moral grounds one day, it still does not seem compatible with the vagaries of the weather, the severities of climate, and the requirements of our daily work.

COSMIC CLOCKS

"We all live on the same cosmic vessel," wrote Dr. Henri Laborit. Our cosmic vessel is the earth, which sails in the interstellar universe, a fact we were not aware of for thousands of years. At a conference in January 1959, Prof. Georgio Piccardi, the director of the Physical Chemistry Institute at the University of Florence, spoke these profound words: "We do not have to send a man into space or even make him leave his own country or his home for him to experience the effects of the cosmos. Man is always in the universe because the universe is everywhere." [1]

The cosmos surrounding us is neither fixed nor void. It is filled with countless particles and waves that reach our globe, a fact unknown until a few decades ago. The atmosphere surrounds the earth with a protective screen. One role of this screen is to supply oxygen for respiration. It also protects us from those forces in the cosmos that are most dangerous to health. Without this atmospheric screen life on earth would be destroyed by the cosmic rays coming from the heart of the universe, or by solar protons, which are as penetrating as X-rays or gamma rays.

But fortunately the screen is not impenetrable. The atmo-

---

1. G. Piccardi, *Phénomènes astrophysiques et événements terrestres,* Convention at the Palais de la Découverte, Paris, January 24, 1959.

sphere does allow light to pass through. Otherwise our earth would constantly be dark, and we would know nothing of the heavens above. It also lets infrared rays penetrate, allowing the gentle warmth of the sun to reach us. Otherwise we would live in an ice age. Without the ultraviolet rays that also penetrate this protective screen, we would not be born, nor could we survive without them.

According to astrophysicists, there are two "windows" in the atmospheric screen. The first allows light, heat, and ultraviolet rays to enter. We have been aware of this "window" for a long time. But the second window, discovered comparatively recently, allows electromagnetic long waves of the frequency of radio waves to pass through. The study of these waves has given birth to a revolutionary new branch of astronomy—radio astronomy. This discovery is also important for medicine. Very long electromagnetic waves influence biological phenomena, as we have seen.

The atmosphere is therefore a selective screen that allows useful rays to enter and rejects or absorbs those which could destroy life on earth. But the "heavens" are not unchanging. Sometimes they experience severe disruption, and then the atmosphere cannot repel all the cosmic invasions. Thus some of the cosmos does succeed in reaching us. It does this either indirectly, by causing atmospheric turbulence which has a vital influence on our health, or directly, by disturbing the major terrestrial factors influencing our biological exchanges, namely electricity and magnetism. That man's body reacts to these forces has been demonstrated only recently.

A New Dimension

The cosmos has many faces, but the sun is the focal point of our solar system. It is the generator of all life on earth, but it could destroy life in an instant. The moon, the planets —in fact the entire galaxy—are more subtle but equally wondrous and disquieting aspects of the cosmic forces acting on us.

A whole new branch of medicine has developed around these influences over the last fifty years. This "cosmic medicine" should not be confused with "space medicine," which deals with the astronauts' physiological reactions and prepares them for landing on the surface of the moon and the planets. The aim of "cosmic medicine" is broader in one sense, yet more limited in another. Cosmic physicians study the influence of the cosmos on each and every one of us living here on earth. But the two branches of medicine, cosmic and spatial, complement each other. They are adding a new dimension to our knowledge of biology. The study of the influence of cosmic phenomena on our health is now a universal pursuit of modern science.

An entire section of the 1966 convention of the International Society of Biometeorology in New Brunswick, New Jersey, was devoted to the discussion of extraterrestrial influences on chemical and biological phenomena. According to Prof. Rémy Chauvin, "Medicine, in its search for knowledge, is now extending its horizons into the domain of meteorology." [2]

Man and the Telephone

During the interval between the two world wars, a doctor from Nice, Maurice Faure, made a perplexing observation. Disruption of the telephone service almost always corresponded to a sudden deterioration in the health of his patients. This was very annoying because it meant that he did not receive emergency calls at the very time his patients

2. *Science et Vie* (December 1958), p. 122.

needed him the most. Once, when this disruption had been particularly severe, he read in the newspaper that there had been a large magnetic storm in the United States that had caused a breakdown in the telephone and telegraph service for several hours.

Puzzled and surprised, Dr. Faure consulted an astronomer, M. Vallot, who explained this strange occurrence to him, "These telephone disruptions are not rare," he said. "The phenomenon that causes this can also cause a compass to start spinning, an aurora borealis to appear, or even earthquakes or volcanic eruptions to occur. It is the sun that is the origin of these disturbances in terrestrial magnetism. For the sun is not that unchanging sphere, that gold coin, glorified by the Pythagoreans. Its surface changes, and spots appear on it periodically. These huge dark areas, formed by immense magnetic vortexes, release fiery waves and particles when they are directed toward earth. They are responsible for the magnetic disturbances we experience on our globe."

"But," said Dr. Faure, "since the human organism is disturbed at the same time as the telephone, this is also the fault of the sun isn't it?"

The two scientists then decided to combine their efforts. And the following story, narrated by Dr. Faure, describes the results of their combined work.

"We decided to work together to see if the occurrence of sunspots coincided with a relapse in some human diseases. Dr. Sardou was invited to participate in the study, and the initial research was performed in the following way. In his observatory on Mount Blanc Mr. Vallot recorded all occurrences of sunspots. At the same time Dr. Sardou recorded the morbid deteriorations he observed in his patients at Nice on the Mediterranean coast, while I recorded those occurring at a health resort in the mountains of central France. We all kept our results to ourselves. But after 267 consecutive days of observation we compared data, and it was easy to affirm that these results were chronologically superimposable. Of the twenty-five sunspots seen, twenty-one had been accompanied by a very distinct general deterioration in health. Later I studied the relationship between sunspots and series of sudden deaths and found that sudden mortalities are twice as numerous when sunspots are present." [3]

Drs. Faure and Sardou and Mr. Vallot reported their observations in a paper presented to the French Academy of Medicine on July 4, 1922. This date is, in some ways, the birth date of cosmic medicine.

Epidemics Every Eleven Years

A Russian historian, A. L. Tchijewsky, who later became a professor at Moscow's School of Medicine, was pursuing similar research at the same time that Dr. Faure was conducting his investigations. An unusual intuition was at the basis of his life's work. As a historian he had access to all his country's archives. Old chronicles related in full detail the greatest scourges of their times—plague, cholera, and typhus epidemics. All these catastrophes were cyclic: they struck suddenly one year, ravaged entire regions, killed thousands of people, then were dormant for several years before striking again.

Tchijewsky decided to correlate these disastrous outbreaks with the cycle of sunspots. The number of sunspots increases for five or six years, at which time it reaches its maximum. Then the number decreases over an equal period of time, eventually reaching a "calm sun" period. Then the cycle begins again.

If we admit that sunspots are capable of influencing our health by modifying meteorological or geophysical conditions, then their effect should be stronger during the periods when their number is at its maximum.

3. Quoted by B. Tocquet, *Cycles et Rythmes*, p. 38.

Tchijewsky spent his whole life collecting, recording, and comparing the dates of Russia's major epidemics, and then those of the entire world. The results of his research are impressive. The great plagues of history, such as cholera and diphtheria in Europe, recurrent typhus in Russia, and smallpox in the United States, all seem to follow faithfully the sun's eleven-year cycle. According to Tchijewsky's works, epidemics tend to occur in years ·of maximum solar activity and are rare during the calm-sun years.[4]

Tchijewsky published many statistical reports in support of his theories. For example, one report on cholera epidemics in the last century in Russia showed that from 1816 to 1900 the epidemics were usually strongest when they coincided with a maximum amount of solar activity. The very significant graphs in Figure IV illustrate epidemics of recurrent typhus in Moscow, smallpox in Chicago, and diphtheria in Russia.

Today major epidemics have almost totally disappeared from civilized countries, thanks to advances in hygiene and especially to the development of vaccines. The third graph in Figure V., concerning smallpox epidemics in Chicago, illustrates the spectacular drop in this disease after the introduction of compulsory vaccinations. The success of these vaccinations has limited the work of Tchijewsky and those continuing in his footsteps. It has become more difficult to study the periodicity of epidemics since 1930. However, some heavily populated countries with poor sanitary conditions, such as India, still provide ample information for the continuation of this research.

The conclusions reached by the Soviet scientist are of practical interest to us. Although medical science has been able to control diseases like typhus, smallpox, and cholera, they still exist in the world and can strike again if conditions conducive to their propagation, such as natural disasters,

4. A. L. Tchijewsky, *L'action de l'activité solaire sur les épidémies* (1934), pp. 1034–41.

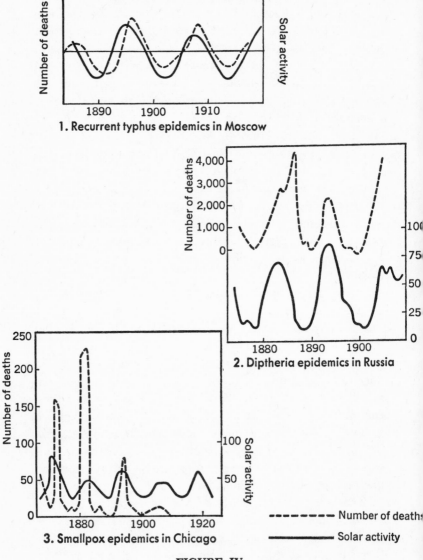

1. Recurrent typhus epidemics in Moscow

2. Diptheria epidemics in Russia

3. Smallpox epidemics in Chicago

---------- Number of deaths

———————— Solar activity

FIGURE IV
SOLAR ACTIVITY AND EPIDEMICS

Whenever solar activity increases, epidemics become more destructive. Solid line: solar activity. Dotted line: number of deaths.

social upheaval, or war, should arise. Since solar cycles can be forecast accurately by astronomers, Tchijewsky's theories, if confirmed, could be a valuable aid in the fight against epidemics. Strict medical surveillance would be necessary when the greatest number of sunspots are occurring. Hopefully, some investigators will verify Tchijewsky's theories and reaffirm his conclusions.

TABLE III

Cholera Epidemics and Solar Activity
(From A. L. Tchijewsky)

| | Solar Activity | |
Maximum of epidemics	Maximum	Minimum
1817	1816	1823
1829–30	1830	1833
1837	1837	1844
1848	1848	1856
1863–66	1860	1867
1870–72	1870	1878
1883–86	1883	1889
1892–94	1894	1900

Virulence of Bacteria

Is there an explanation for the relationship between epidemics and sunspots? In his microbiology laboratory in Germany, Prof. H. Bortels performed countless experiments on the activity and virulence of bacteria. He has been able to prove that bacterial activity is related to solar activity.

Furthermore, all great migrations of animals seem to follow certain rhythms that are strangely linked to the sun's cycle. One Soviet entomologist, Tcherbinovsky, mapped the invasion routes of grasshoppers throughout the world for forty years in order to see if solar activity affected their proliferation. Derjavine, his fellow-countryman, studied sturgeon in the Caspian Sea and discovered that these fish proliferate, then die in vast quantities following the eleven-year cycle of sunspots.

According to entomologists, migrations are the result of abnormal proliferation of a race, a sort of mass cancer. This anarchic proliferation is similar to the sudden multiplication of bacteria in a test tube. The following theory has been advanced to explain Tchijewsky's findings that certain solar and geomagnetic phenomena cause bacteria which have been dormant for several years to suddenly become virulent and this results in an epidemic. On the other hand if Faure and Sardou are correct, then man's resistance decreases when increased solar activity occurs. So at the very time that man is most susceptible, bacteria are most virulent, and this relationship permits epidemics to occur. These theories have yet to be scientifically proven.

Solar Eruptions and Infarctions

At a medical meeting in March 1958, a French doctor, J. Poumailloux, together with a meteorologist, Mr. Viart, presented a very unusual report. They stated that myocardial infarctions do not occur at random, but seem determined by very precise solar coordinates. Whenever a sudden disturbance occurs on the sun, there seems to be a response in our blood vessels and arteries causing blood clots to form in those individuals predisposed to clotting. These clots can obstruct the coronary arteries and cause an infarction.

The two researchers cited the year 1957 as an example. During that year they observed an increase in the number of infarctions between January 17 and January 22. They recorded no infarctions in April or July, but there was another large increase from September 1 to September 3. Solar activity, which had generally been moderate that year, suddenly increased from January 17 to January 25 and from August 28 to September 3.[5]

The Incident on May 17, 1959

A highly exceptional solar phenomenon occurred on May 17, 1959. It was observed throughout the whole world, but with special interest in the U.S.S.R. On May 17 alone, the observatory of the Soviet Academy of Sciences recorded the appearance of three powerful solar eruptions. These occurred at 5:24 A.M., 5:45 A.M., and 7:06 A.M. Moving at a speed of 10,000 miles per second, the torrent ejected from the sun reached the earth the next day on May 18.

Located on the edge of the Black Sea are the Sochi clinics, where Soviet patients are often sent to convalesce. N. V. Romensky, the city's health director, reported that on May 18 the number of cardiovascular emergencies there suddenly increased to twenty whereas there were usually only two per day. This is a tenfold increase.

Professor Romensky had already made similar observations at Sochi in 1956. At that time the number of cardiovascular emergencies tripled during the months of February and August, when strong solar eruptions occurred.[6]

At a meeting of geophysicists and meteorologists in Ottawa, Canada, in April 1960, Professor Giordano from Italy reported the results of his analysis of myocardial infarctions between 1954 and 1958. Solar activity was on the increase during those years, and Professor Giordano observed a parallel augmentation in the number of infarctions occurring

5. J. Poumailloux and R. Viart, "Corrélations possibles entre l'incidence des infarctus du myocarde et l'augmentation des activités solaire et géomagnétique," *Bull. Acad. Méd.*, Vol. 143, nos. 7–8 (1959), p. 167.

6. N. V. Romensky, *Collection of Scientific Works from the Administration of the Thermal and Climatic Health Clinics* (Sochi, 1960).

in his community. They increased from 200 in 1954 to 450 in 1958. Giordano gave a detailed day-by-day analysis of the cardiac emergencies. He found that there were days when there were a great number of infarctions, and furthermore, that on those days, geomagnetic storms caused by sudden variations in solar activity had occurred. This confirms the observations made by Poumailloux and Viart.

Aurora Borealis and Hemorrhages

In 1934 two German investigators, G. and B. Düll, compiled some comprehensive statistics on the distribution of deaths from tuberculosis on or close to days characterized by strong solar eruptions. The graph in Figure V summarizes some of their results. It represents the number of deaths from tuberculosis in Hamburg during the year 1936. The "O" day represents days on which solar eruptions occurred. On these days, the number of deaths is distinctly greater than ten days before and ten days after.[7]

At about the same time in Argentina Dr. Puig noted that pulmonary hemorrhages were more frequent whenever the local observatory recorded magnetic storms. On calm days only 1 or 2 percent of the patients in his hospital had hemorrhages. But during periods of magnetic disturbance this percentage rose to 10 and 13 percent.

During the past thirty years this topic has often been discussed in medical journals, occasionally with contradictory conclusions. In 1953 Professor Helmut Berg, of Cologne, Germany, could find no connection between sudden pulmonary emboli and solar storms. But another German doctor, O. Lingemann, undertook to study all the medical documents from West Germany's sanatoria. He was struck by a curious

7. H. Berg, *Solarterrestrische Beziehungen in Meteorologie und Biologie* (Leipzig, 1957), p. 131.

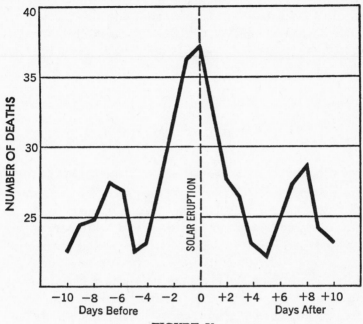

NUMBER OF DEATHS

SOLAR ERUPTION

−10 −8 −6 −4 −2 0 +2 +4 +6 +8 +10
Days Before   Days After

FIGURE V
SOLAR ERUPTIONS AND NUMBER OF DEATHS
FROM TUBERCULOSIS

There are more deaths on days when solar eruptions occur (day 0) than on those days preceding or following these eruptions (Hamburg 1936).[8]

phenomenon. During the four years of his research, from 1948 to 1952, German observatories had recorded eighteen aurorae borealis, a very rare phenomenon in Germany. By comparing their dates with his medical records, Dr. Lingemann discovered that the days on which the aurorae borealis had occurred had been very dramatic in the sanatoria. The doctors had had to take care of many more cases of hemoptysis than usual. The aurora borealis is caused by strong solar activity that disturbs the atmosphere's upper strata. The intense ionization of the air causes the multicolored streamers

8. *Ibid.*

of the aurora borealis, one of nature's grander spectacles. Here again atmospheric disturbances caused by excessive solar activity seem to be a danger signal for tubercular patients.[9]

Precautionary Measures

Naturally all these results can only be considered as statistical tendencies. They imply no fixed rules. They are, above all, a warning signal. On days when there are magnetic storms caused by solar activity, we should, when possible, try to limit our activities, smoke less tobacco, and avoid overexcitement and fatigue, because all these factors affect the blood constituents and therefore favor either blood clotting or hemorrhage, according to the individual's predisposition. Solar disturbances risk provoking a latent crisis in some susceptible subjects.

Fortunately, the doctor is not helpless before these cosmic upheavals that affect our bodies. Effective preventive measures have been introduced, such as those pioneered by Professor Romensky in the Sochi clinics. He keeps in constant contact with astronomical observatories and takes special precautions as soon as the astronomers report any increase in solar activity. He has built Faraday cages to protect his most susceptible patients from the dangerous rays, and he gives them more intensive therapeutic treatment during these stormy periods. These revolutionary measures have considerably reduced the number of cardiac and pulmonary emergencies among his patients.

9. O. Lingemann, "Tuberkulöses Lungenbluten und meteorologische Einflüsse seit Einführung der Chemotherapie," Der Tuberkulosearzt, No. 9 (1955), p. 261.

Blood Changes

How can catastrophic events occurring on the sun have such a disastrous effect on our health? Poumailloux and Viart define the problem: "We still have .to discover the mechanism which causes the human organism, or at least certain predisposed organisms, to react unfavorably to increased solar and geomagnetic activity. If an infarction is caused by a coronary obstruction following an abrupt increase in coagulation time *in situ,* it seems that there should be a parallel increase in the number of cases of phlebitis and other intravascular coagulative complaints. Hematologists working in the blood-transfusion service of Saint-Antoine Hospital (Paris) have pointed out that spontaneous and apparently inexplicable variations in coagulation tests occur at certain times, even in normal subjects. Similarly, all phthisiologists have observed the temporary increase in hemoptysis at certain periods. It is difficult to see how blood constituency could be influenced by external geophysical factors unless it is through the intermediary of the hormonal and autonomic nervous systems." [10]

The reactions of healthy individuals to these external influences proved to be the key for discovering the cause of pathological manifestations. Rivolier pointed out one of the most intriguing biological effects. "On some days, at certain times, every blood test performed on healthy subjects shows the same type of deviation when analyzed. This deviation is independent of the subject himself, since it occurs in all subjects and can only be associated with an outside event, namely a cosmic event." [11]

This cosmic event has a marked influence on our blood. The sun's vagaries are capable of greatly modifying the leu-

10. Poumailloux and Viart, *op. cit.,* p. 167.
11. Rivolier, *op cit.,* p. 61.

cocyte (or white-blood-cell) count of healthy subjects. For example, during the great solar eruption of February 1956, some precise blood counts were made in the Soviet Union. A large number of the subjects examined showed leukopenia, which is an abnormal decrease in the number of white blood cells. Before the solar eruption only 14 percent of the total Soviet population had leukopenia with fewer than 5,000 leukocytes per cubic millimeter of blood. This percentage doubled after the solar eruption, reaching 29 percent. One month later, in March, it dropped again to 13 percent. By July it was only 12 percent and by October, 11 percent.

Too Many White Blood Cells

Occasionally an abnormal increase of certain blood constituents is noted rather than a diminution. Nicholas Schultz, a Soviet hematologist, reported that in 1957 and 1958 doctors were puzzled by a constant increase in the incidence of lymphocytosis. Lymphocytosis is characterized by an increase in the number of white blood cells called lymphocytes.[12] Doctors remembered that at the end of the World War I a similar phenomenon had been observed. A German specialist, Dr. Klieneberger, had even termed it "lymphocytosis of war." War and famine were believed responsible for it. Then the cases of lymphocytosis diminished. However, there had been no war or famine in western Europe when lymphocytosis increased once again. Excessive use of sulfa drugs and antibiotics was blamed. But these drugs had not been discovered in 1917. Neither they nor famine and war could be responsible for the periodic recurrence of large numbers of cases of lymphocytosis.

The only plausible explanation is solar activity. In 1917

12. N. Schultz, "Lymphocytoses relatives et activité solaire," *Revue Médicale de Nancy* (June 1961).

and 1957 solar activity was passing through a peak phase. This fact has been confirmed by Soviet investigators. Under the direction of Dr. N. Schultz they performed thousands of blood tests on normal subjects and compared the results regularly with the activity of the sun. They obtained an almost perfect parallel between the percentage of cases of lymphocytosis and the increase in solar activity published monthly by astronomers. Figure VI represents one of Dr. Schultz's many observations for the year 1957.

A Living Sun Dial

The white blood cells are not the only blood constituents affected. All components of the blood are sensitive to the effects of the cosmos. M. Takata, a biologist from Tokyo, became famous through his discoveries on blood serum. After developing a chemical procedure called "Takata's reaction," which analyzed the albumin of the blood, he went on in 1938 to discover disproportionate changes in the blood-serum levels. These changes were synchronous throughout the entire world wherever Takata's reaction was being used. The agent causing these changes was influencing subjects over the entire globe simultaneously. Takata concluded that if the phenomenon was worldwide, the cause had to be cosmic. After twenty years of research he was able to establish a specific close relationship between blood serum and various solar manifestations such as sunrise, eruptions, the eleven-year cycle, etc. It is Takata who says: "Man is a living sun dial." [14]

Doctors know that the blood of healthy people is continually changing. These changes depend on age, fatigue, the time of meals, etc. But now physicians have to take a new

14. M. Takata: "Ueber eine neue biologisch wirksame Komponente der Sonnenstrahlung," *Archiv. Met. Geophys. Bioklimat,* B (1951), p. 486.

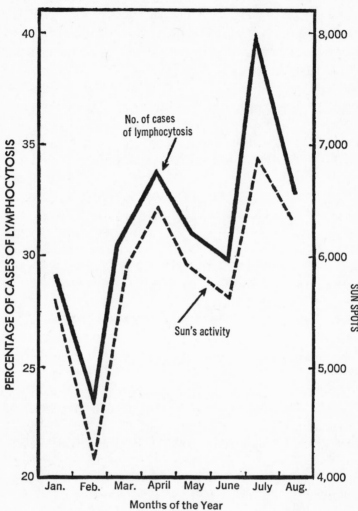

FIGURE VI
SUNSPOTS AND WHITE BLOOD CELLS

From January to August 1957 the incidence of lymphocytosis in healthy subjects increased and decreased paralleling the sun's activity, which was measured by the number of sunspots.[13]

13. N. Schultz, Les Globules blancs de sujets bien portants et les taches solaires, Toulouse Medical, no. 10 (1960), p. 741.

variable into consideration: the solar variable, responsible for great fluctuations in blood values. *These modifications are normal.* They represent a healthy organism's adaptation to environmental influences. Medical science has discovered that in order to avoid diagnostic errors, allowances must be made for these fluctuations.

A Bright Light

The fact that a healthy subject's blood can be so sensitive to solar fluctuations throws light on the origin of pulmonary and cardiovascular disorders observed in patients suffering from these illnesses or predisposed to them. Rivolier very accurately wrote: "The blood's cellular and physico-chemical composition reflects various functions of the organism in terms of its role as a vehicle and intermediary between the various organs. This explains why medicine can analyze some constant factors of the blood to determine any abnormal function that may correspond to changes found in the blood analysis." [15]

The composition of the blood is dependent upon our organism's blood-producing organs: spleen, bone marrow, etc. If the blood's composition is affected, then other physiological functions, such as the functioning of the endocrine glands and the nervous system, can be affected too. There are plenty of medical observations where solar influences appear to have an important effect on physiological mechanisms.

Cosmos and Eclampsia

Eclampsia is a serious disturbance that can develop in women late in pregnancy. It is characterized by convulsions

15. J. Rivolier, *op cit.*, p. 61.

that appear quite similar to epileptic convulsions. Mild eclampsia usually responds to treatment. However, severe forms can result in coma and death.

From their daily experience obstetricians and midwives have long been aware that eclampsia occurs "in waves" and have thought the weather responsible for it. In 1942 two German doctors, E. Bach and L. Schluck, decided to make a scientific study of the problem. They observed sudden flare-ups of eclampsia in maternity wards. But weather changes, long considered the cause, did not play the major role. The sun's influence was generally the determining factor. Calm-sun days did not provoke episodes of eclampsia; such episodes tended to occur during periods of increased solar activity.[16]

This disease, if diagnosed in time, responds rapidly to appropriate treatment. Bach and Schluck have suggested that astronomers should keep obstetricians informed of approaching solar storms. Obstetricians can guard their patients more closely and so reduce the threat of eclampsia and its sequelae for future mothers.

Outbreaks of Violence

In 1965 there were more than 12,000 highway deaths in France, and more than 200,000 automobile accidents. The death toll increases by 10 percent every year, but statistics have shown that only one-third of these accidents are due to mechanical failures. In two out of three cases, human error (incompetence, negligence, bad judgment) is to blame.

On some days there are many more accidents than on others. Highway-control authorities know that there are

16. E. Bach and L. Schluck, "Untersuchungen über den Einfluss von meteorologischen, ionosphärischen und solaren Faktoren, sowie der Mondphasen auf die Auslösung von Eklampsie," *Zentralblatt für Gynäkologie*, 66 (1942), p. 196.

"black weekends" when fatalities pile up along the roadside while other weekends are relatively accident-free.

Even more serious is the fact that at certain times (January 1965 is an example) some drivers who are involved in only minor accidents suddenly become very aggressive:

"A North African leaves his car and shoots another driver in the head. . . ." "Violent driver punches a man to death. . . ." "A young driver strikes a pedestrian crossing at a crosswalk, slaps a woman who tries to intervene, and then disappears." Then the outburst of violent incidents ceases as suddenly as it started.

Psychologists and doctors have long tried to determine the motivation for such incredible behavior. This is not easy because there are many causes. In January 1965 several were suggested: excitation from New Year's celebrations, excessive intake of alcohol, the illusion of being on vacation followed by a return to work after too short a rest, the bad weather, etc. All of these factors can change *Homo sapiens*, once in his automobile, into an incompetent driver or a murderer.

Some authorities have suggested that in addition to these very terrestrial and human causes there may be a cosmic cause. Could solar eruptions reaching our planet act either directly or indirectly on our nervous system just as they act on our cardiovascular system? This is a significant question.

A German meteorologist, R. Reiter, studied this problem statistically in 1952. He patiently researched the dates and times of 130,000 road accidents that had occurred in Bavaria and the principal cities of Germany and Austria. His results showed a 10 percent increase in the accident rate on days following solar eruptions.

R. Martini, another German researcher, compared industrial accidents with solar activity. He eliminated massive disasters (such as the collapse of large structures, gas explosions in mines, or the bursting of dams). He considered only accidents caused by clumsiness, inattention, or nervous irritation on the part of the workers. His statistics cover 306 working days in the Ruhr coal mines during which time 5,580 accidents occurred. In Dr. Martini's opinion, the results of his study are quite conclusive: miners have more accidents when strong magnetic disturbances occur in the atmosphere. There are relatively few accidents on calm days.[17]

Doctor Martini believes that magnetic storms disturb and retard the workmen's reactions. Moreover, laboratory studies show that reaction speeds are slower during magnetic storms.

The Sun and Mental Diseases

Some investigators believe the sun can cause nervous disorders even more distinctive than the previously described

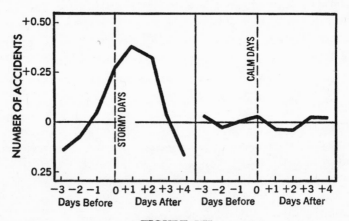

FIGURE VII
THE SUN AND ACCIDENTS

In the Ruhr coal mines the accident rate is much higher on magnetically stormy days (left graph) than on magnetically calm days (right graph).[18]

17. R. Martini: "Der Einfluss der Sonnentätigkeit auf die Häufung von Unfälilen," *Zentralblatt Arbeitsmedizin u. Arbeitschurtz*, 2 (1952), p. 98.

18. H. Berg, *Solar-terrestrische Beziehungen in Meteorologie und Biologie* (Leipzig, 1957), p. 136.

aberrations. Father Moreux, former director of the Bourges observatory, wrote in 1930: "The electric flow emanating from the sun acts on our nervous system, and I have often observed that many people, especially children, are more irritable during phases of increased solar activity. Teachers have to administer more punishments when there are magnetic storms caused by solar disturbances. In some subjects these unconscious influences cause nervousness. In other sickly people complex consequences such as breathing difficulties, attacks of gout or rheumatism, migraine, neuralgia, and even fits of anger appear." Some investigators consider that any classification attributing all these varying effects to the sun is much too rigid.

Nevertheless, in 1963 an article in the English scientific journal *Nature*, written by three psychiatrists from the New York Veterans' Hospital, H. Friedman, R. Becker, and C. Bachman, reported an amazing parallel between the number of patients admitted to New York's psychiatric hospitals and terrestrial magnetic disturbances.

How could these disturbances cause a reaction in the cerebrum of a mental patient? Dr. Becker stated: "Subtle changes in the intensity of the geomagnetic field can affect the nervous system by altering the living organism's own electromagnetic field." He located areas on the human body with positive electrical charges and areas with negative electrical charges. Contact with waves bearing a different charge disturbs these areas. In some cases the patient even faints. By experimenting in his laboratory, Dr. Becker was able to change the electroencephalographic brain-wave tracings of animals exposed to intense magnetic fields.[19]

19. H. Friedman, R. Becker, and C. Bachman, "Geomagnetic Parameters and Psychiatric Hospital Admission," *Nature*, 200 (1963), p. 626.

Extenuating Circumstances?

In addition to the restlessness of mental patients, G. and B. Düll, the two German researchers previously mentioned, made a survey of 24,739 suicides in Germany, Switzerland, and Denmark, and discovered an increase in the incidence of nervous depression and suicide when there is intense solar activity.

The Soviet professor Tchijewsky believed that social changes, economic crises, and wars could be partially influenced by important solar activity. This opinion seems rather extreme, and there is insufficient evidence to support it. More direct determining factors of an economic and psychological nature can better explain these all-too-human events.

But this strange observation by the same scientist is worthy of mention: "The time will come when a judge who has to pass judgment on an accused person will demand the pertinent astronomical and meteorological conditions prevailing when the crime was committed. If the crime took place at a time when sunspots were reaching their maximum intensity, the defendant will be held less responsible for his crime." Obviously science and justice must wait for scientific proof before applying this theory. But one day . . . who knows? Perhaps we shall actually see meteorologists giving evidence in court along with toxicologists and medical experts.

The Moon and Atmospheric Conditions

For a long time scientists denied the possibility of the moon's influence on man. Their instruments indicated nothing to show a physical influence of the moon on our planet other than its influence on tides.

During the International Geophysical Year in 1966 it was shown that the moon, like the sun, can modify the earth's magnetic state. Data collected by artificial satellites and, more recently, by instruments placed on the moon's surface are replacing old sayings with scientific facts. We now know, for instance, that the moon can deflect and alter solar winds, those clouds of protons from solar storms that affect the earth's magnetic fields.

Since the dawn of history man has believed that the moon influences the weather. "The weather changes with the moon" is still a popular saying meaning that changes of weather are determined by the four phases of the moon. At the end of last century, students at France's War College were taught to use the moon as a basis for weather forecasting. The method was known as Bugeaud's Law, named after Marshal Bugeaud, who taught there. Marshal Bugeaud was not the inventor of this formula, merely an exponent of it. He is said to have learned it from a monk in a monastery in Spain. This is the best-known version of the law: "The weather during the whole lunar month will be like the fifth day, eleven times out of twelve, unless the weather changes on the sixth day." [20] During the Algerian campaigns of the 1840s Marshal Bugeaud used this rule to decide on which days to move his troops. However, fifty years later when General Delcambre, the Director of National Meteorology, tried to prove Bugeaud's law scientifically, he was unable to do so.

Does the moon have any influence on the weather? Legends often contain a grain of truth. In 1962 meteorologists D. Bradley, M. Woodbury, and G. Brier published a comprehensive statistical survey in the American Journal *Science*, indicating that very rainy days tend to occur during the moon's first and third quarters.[21] Two Australian scientists,

20. P. Saintyves: *L'Astrologie populaire* (Popular Astrology, 1937 p. 56).
21. D. Bradley, M. Woodbury, and G. Brier, "Lunar Synodical Period and Widespread Precipitation," *Science*, 147 (1962), p. 748.

Adderly and Bowen, have confirmed these results. No clear explanation for this phenomenon, which seems to justify ancient beliefs, has yet been given. But it does appear that the moon exerts an influence on meteorological phenomena. Two French meteorologists, V. Mironovitch and R. Viart, after extensive studies, explained the moon's role in certain types of weather called "blocking." They can predict long-term atmospheric changes by evaluating the relative positions of the sun, the earth, and the moon in space.[22]

The Moon and Crops

The appearance of a red moon in the spring, the "April moon," has always been dreaded by farmers. Many sayings illustrate dangers: "Frosts brought by the April moon stop plants from growing"; "When the April moon has passed, there are no more frosts to fear."

It is a fact that the April moon is often accompanied by late frosts that are very harmful to crops. François Arago, a physicist, has shown that the moon itself is not responsible for this damage. When the moon appears rust-colored, it is because the atmosphere is too pure, causing a rapid chilling of the air. This frosty air, colder than usual, can injure the young plants.

Farmers maintain that the lunar cycle influences the growth of some plants, particularly vegetables. It is a fact that plants do follow certain lunar rhythms. But Reinberg and Ghata have pointed out that rhythms are primarily evident in marine algae or aquatic plants, and that the lunar influence seems to act only indirectly on these plants through the tides.

22. V. Mironovitch and R. Viart, *Interruption du courant zonal en Europe occidentale et sa liaison avec l'activité solaire*, Section de recherche de la Société Centrale d'Etudes et d'Applications Météorologiques, Paris.

Is the moon's influence on plants an imaginary one? Not according to Frank A. Brown and his colleagues at Northwestern University, who have shown that the oxygen consumption of numerous plants varies throughout the month and the lunar day. The growth of plants is closely related to their oxygen needs.

The Moon and Menstruation

The correspondence between the average length of a woman's menstrual cycle and the time it takes the moon to complete a revolution around the earth has intrigued man throughout the ages. Even the word menstruate is derived etymologically from the lunar month. Why is the menstrual cycle a twenty-eight day cycle, about the same length of time as the moon's?

Many scientists considered this more than a mere coincidence; they saw it as a cause-and-effect relationship. Physicians often felt that the moon did exert an influence on the female cycle. In a collective work on rhythms published in 1944 Dr. H. Duprat wrote: "The first menstruation of a normal healthy woman occurs when the moon is at the same position in the zodiac as when she was born. Provided that the woman remains healthy, the same function should recur under similar circumstances." The scientific basis of such statements is not readily apparent and, of course, must be verified statistically.

Gynecologist D. L. Gunn's research is a model of scientific precision. In order to obtain completely objective material for his analysis, he asked all his patients to send him a postcard with their name on it when their menses started. The date would be verified by the postmark. Gunn collected 10,000 postcards before beginning his analysis. But he received no reward for his labor; he could discover no relationship between the lunar cycle and the days when women started to menstruate every month.[23]

Other researchers who have studied the question obtained no positive results either. In 1951 a German doctor, H. Hosemann, compiled a complete list of all the studies previously published on this topic. The list decidedly weakens the belief in a correlation between the moon and menstruation. Hosemann was unable to find any connection after analyzing more than 15,000 cases.

It seems, therefore, that no particular moment of the lunar month provokes menstruation. But can we be sure that the moon plays no role? Those believing in the moon's influence feel that more subtle studies should be undertaken, and they make a good point for their case. Perhaps some women are more receptive at a given moment of the lunar month than others. Would it not be preferable to follow a series of cases individually for several years rather than compile enormous quantities of statistics from all over the world, which might conceal numerous different patterns.

Other gynecologists who oppose the moon theory point out that it is very rare for a woman's menstrual cycle to be regular. It varies according to season, age, and state of health. Many biologists also reject the moon theory because the menstrual cycle of other female mammals is not the same length as a lunar month. For female chimpanzees the cycle lasts thirty-six days, for cows twenty days, for guinea pigs fifteen days, etc., all of which are far from our twenty-eight-day lunar cycle. Biologists reject the dangerously anthropomorphic opinion that our species is the only mammal species in which the moon influences the female menstrual cycle.

23. D. L. Gunn et al., "Menstrual Periodicity: Statistical Observation on a Large Sample of Normal Cases," J. Obstetr. Gynaecol., 44 (1937), p. 839.

A Great Midwife?

"During the period of the full moon deliveries are believed to be easier," wrote Plutarch. In the sixteenth century a famous doctor, A. Mizault, wrote in the flowery style of that time: "When the moon is rich in light and consequently at the height of its powers (full moon), it liberally communicates this strength to the female sex by spontaneously breaking her waters and starting uterine contractions. This it does through harmony and friendship, which it has stored with Mother Nature." [24]

But once again we must disappoint the propounders of these moon theories. Recently three Frenchmen, Prof. A. Duchateau, Professor Roblot, and Dr. J. Meyer, and a German, Dr. R. Reiter, showed that deliveries are equally distributed throughout the four lunar quarters with no obvious trends observed during any one of the four phases.

In the sixteenth century Bacon wrote: "It is possible that children and young cattle born during a full moon are larger and stronger than those born during the waning phase." [25] It is very unlikely that this is true, and doctors certainly no longer believe it.

Inhabitants of the islands of the North Sea maintain that the moon is a great midwife. They claim that more children are born when the tides are rising than when they are ebbing. K. W. Schultze, a doctor on Norderney Island off the German coast, tried to confirm this belief. He studied the island's birth register and noted all the births that had occurred during rising tides and all those that had occurred during ebbing tides. He found exactly the same number in both cases. The moon therefore does not intervene. Dr. Schultz, however, has no illusions. He wrote: "My observa-

24. A. Mizault, *Les Secrets de la Lune*, p. 5.
25. Francis Bacon, *Works*, Vol. I (London, 1750), p. 187.

tions will not stop the island's midwife from calmly telling the anxious expectant father, 'We have plenty of time. Your child won't be born until the tide comes in.'" [26]

However, Dr. H. Kirchhoff from Leipzig noted that many deliveries occur right at high tide, the time when the moon is passing its highest or lowest point.

At the beginning of the century Svente Arrhenius, a Swedish scientist and winner of a Nobel Prize, studied 25,000 individuals and found a correlation between the maximum number of births and a specific moment in the lunar cycle. "He tried," wrote Reinberg and Ghata, "to link this fact to a correlation between the length and date of menstruation, namely the date of the last period before pregnancy began. Arrhenius admitted that the deciding factor could be variations in atmospheric electricity, whose twenty-seven-to-thirty-two-day cycle corresponds to the lunar cycle." [27] This possibility has yet to be fully explored.

The Sex of Children

Is the moon able to determine a child's sex? Legend claims this to be true. Casanova relates an amusing story along these lines in his *Memoirs*. One of his many conquests was jealous of him. Casanova replied with the assurance of a seducer who has never been rejected, "I shall prove to you that I love only you, if you will allow me to spend two hours tonight in your arms."

"That is impossible. My husband has learned that the moon is changing today."

"But does he need the moon's permission to fulfill such sweet obligations toward you?"

---

26. K. W. Schultze, "Beeinflussen Flut und Ebbe den Geburtseintritt?" *Deutsche Medizinische Wochenschrift* (1949), p. 311.
27. Reinberg and Ghata, *op. cit.*, p. 50.

"According to his beliefs in astrology, this is the way to preserve his health and to have a son, if the heavens choose to grant him one."

"I was obliged to wait," concluded Casanova.

P. Saintyves found many examples of this in his collection of popular beliefs about the moon: "If a woman conceives during a waxing moon, her child will be of the stronger sex: but if she conceives during a waning moon, then the child will be a girl. Boys are born in the first quarter and girls in the waning phase, as girls are born during a new moon and boys during the last quarter. And finally, when a child is going to be born in the final quarter, people 'know' in advance that it will be a boy.[28]

There are even more complex beliefs. It used to be claimed that the sex of an unborn child could be predicted if it was known in which phase of the moon the previous child had been born. In an old English memoir written three centuries ago a letter from a man to a member of his family states: "My wife fortunately has given birth to a boy thanks to the moon's quarter. The next child should also be a boy."

These beliefs are poetic and quaint, but hardly well-founded. Dr. Hosemann's clear, precise statistics have convinced doctors that there are no specific days of the lunar month for producing boys or girls. There are so many theories on how the moon can exercise such an influence that one becomes lost in them. Geneticists have proven that the sex of a child is due to chance and is determined at the time of conception.

Diseases and Deaths Related to the Moon

Since it is often believed that certain phases of the moon facilitate childbirth, it is likewise felt that there are some

28. P. Saintyves, *L'Astrologie populaire* (1937), p. 211.

phases during which mortality increases. In his book *Temperaments* R. Allendy mentions the observations he made at a sanatorium on the Mediterranean: "We have found that the greatest incidence of hemoptysis and attacks of fever in tuberculous patients occurred from the first quarter to the full moon and that the lowest incidence occurred from full moon to the last quarter. Proportionally the distribution was twelve cases during the former period to one case in the latter. The remaining two lunar phases both present the same frequency, namely about three or four cases per phase."

Today such observations are unconvincing to medical experts. However, a recent *Journal of the Florida Medical Association* carried an article by an American surgeon, Edson J. Andrews, who referred to the cycles of the moon in connection with the causes of excessive post-operative bleeding. He is convinced that the moon plays a decisive role in these hemorrhages. His study showed the danger to be greatest when the moon is full and least at the new moon. He could find no explanation for this. "But," he said, "I am so convinced that I do not hesitate to check the sky. Whenever possible I operate only on dark nights, saving the moonlit nights for romance." [29]

In 1961 a German researcher, Hilman Heckert, found significant relationships between lunar phases and various phenomena such as mortality rates, pneumonia, and uric-acid levels. But these findings have never been confirmed.

Out of this wealth of empirical observations, which are significant? All we can say is that they are all worthy of further investigation using modern scientific methods.

29. Darrell Huff, *Cycles in Your Life* (1965), p. 114.

Full Moon Murderers

Since the beginning of mankind the moon has been credited with a disastrous influence on mental stability so that the word "lunatic" has become synonymous with "mentally deranged." In fact, some believe that repeated crimes by some mentally unbalanced people coincide in a vague way with the moon's phases. Among the most notorious cases cited are those of Doris Gloss, the murderess from Menlo Park, California, and John Edward Allen, the Vampire of Lancashire.

But the mentally disturbed person most often associated with the moon is the "full-moon murderer." The infamous Jack the Ripper was said to be one. So was (or still is?) the Carmes District Murderer, for whom the police are still searching. This man mutilated and killed three tramps during full-moon nights in 1963 and 1964 in the city of Toulouse, France. Police believe that the murderer is a maniac who is compelled to murder by some irresistible force.

It is always difficult to separate truth from sensationalism when evaluating such murders. Does the full moon have such a distinct effect on mentally unbalanced persons? Does its light act as a sort of stimulant for an insane criminal? We often sleep badly when the moon is full in a clear sky and the curtains remain undrawn.

Not long ago, Inspector Wilfred Faust of the Philadelphia Police Department published a report entitled *Effects of Full Moon on Human Behavior*. This report states: "The seventy police officers who deal with telephone complaints claim that they have much more work when the full moon draws near. People whose antisocial behavior has psychotic roots—

as firebugs, kleptomaniacs, destructive drivers, and homicidal alcoholics—seem to go on a rampage more often when the moon is waxing than when it wanes." [30]

Psychiatric Opinions

Are the Philadelphia police officers deluded? Psychiatrists tend to think so because they do not really accept the theory of the moon's influence on criminals. Insane criminals, they say, are manic-depressives like most insane persons. They regularly pass through periods of excitation and periods of depression and dejection. These states can recur at fixed intervals. It is therefore possible that a mental patient who experienced his acute crisis during the full moon will have another crisis during the next full moon. But it is only by chance that this crisis coincides with the full moon. There is no direct link between the moon and mental illness.

But nature is always more complex than we think. It was recently discovered that atmospheric ionization and terrestrial magnetism vary with the lunar phases. Could this interplay of atoms and electrons overstimulate insane criminals? It is now possible to make scientific measurements instead of relying on "impressions," as was previously the case. This is what Leonard J. Ravitz tried to do in 1960 when he measured the differences in electrical potential between the heads and chests of some of his mental patients. The difference changed from day to day according to moon phases and the agitated state of the patient, or so Dr. Ravitz believed. He proposed an original theory to explain this: "The moon does not directly determine human behavior, but by altering the balance of electromagnetic forces of the universe, it is capable of

30. Huff, *op. cit.*, p. 113.

provoking catastrophic consequences in mentally unbalanced subjects." [31]

Up to 1908 the inmates of Bethlehem Hospital were beaten at certain lunar periods as a prophylaxis against violence. In other hospitals the procedures were less systematic but just as harsh. Today less severe and more effective preventive measures have been instituted. But do the new facts justify the old myths about the mentally ill? Only the accumulation of more precise data will enlighten us.

Our Fellow Creatures

Once again we can further our knowledge by observing our fellow creatures. Along the Mediterranean shores it is believed that marine animals such as sea urchins, oysters, and mollusks are fatter at full moon and thinner at new moon. This idea seems based solely on a gross analogy between the moon's apparent size and the size of these animals. However, Prof. Frank A. Brown of Northwestern University decided to investigate these oddities and undertook some unusual experiments. "The fiddler crab, so called because of its violin-shaped claws, changes color in accordance with a lunar rhythm even when it is enclosed in a totally dark room. Rats in their cages are restless when the moon is below the horizon and calm when it rises in the sky. No wall, no matter how thick, can stop this rodent from knowing when the moon is rising or setting." [32]

Other biologists have observed lunar rhythms in the lives of countless living creatures. Take the hatching of mosquitoes, the opening of oyster valves, the egg-laying habits of

31. L. J. Ravitz, "Periodic Changes in Electromagnetic Fields," Ann. N.Y. Acad. of Sciences, 98 (1960), p. 1181.

32. F. A. Brown, "Exogenous Timing of Rat Spontaneous Activity Periods," *Proc. Soc. Exper. Biol. Med.*, 101 (1959), p. 457.

sea urchins. Groups of monkeys are in some mysterious way aware of lunar eclipses. When the moon is lost from view as it is shadowed by the earth, these animals leave their shelter. They appear nervous, huddle against each other, and stand silent and motionless. What wakens them from their sleep? No one yet knows.

Legend is yielding to the scientific search for truth where the effects of the moon are concerned. There is no doubt that many influences, still undiscovered, do emanate from the moon. Scientists are trying to uncover them, but it will take effort. The influences discovered by scientific methods will often have only a remote connection with the legends our forefathers believed. Nevertheless, they will be just as fascinating.

Cosmos and Temperament

As we have seen, atmospheric conditions can be experienced differently according to our individual temperaments. This is equally valid for the effects of the cosmos. Each of us reacts in his own way to cosmic influences. Consider, for example, the effect of the sun's rays on our skin. Two people expose their bodies to the sun's rays, side by side on the same beach for the same length of time. One is olive-skinned and the other is fair-skinned. When they return indoors, one will be tanned and the other will probably be sunburned. This is a typical example of different individual sensitivity to the same cosmic action. It is due to different hereditary constitutions.

We are all familiar with such examples. But cosmic medicine has shown in recent years that the amazing human organism can be influenced by more subtle, undetected factors than the sun's ultraviolet rays. There are lunar and planetary influences in particular that accelerate the progress of childbirth in terms of our heredity. This author has been doing statistical research on this subject for fifteen years.

Planetary Heredity

A survey covering 100,000 births has shown that infants have a heritary predisposition to be born under the same cosmic conditions that prevailed at the birth of their parents. This hereditary action is manifested during the earth's daily rotation on its own axis. When children are born, the other planets of the solar system that are closest to earth—namely the moon, Venus, Mars, Jupiter, and Saturn—occupy positions in the sky similar to the ones they occupied when the parents were born.

Children primarily tend to be born when one of these planets is rising or reaching its highest point in the sky, if this same planet was in the same part of the sky when either of the parents was born. If this "effect of planetary heredity" is to be realized, the baby must obviously have a natural birth. If delivery is artificially induced, either surgically or by the administration of drugs, this relationship does not exist, and the heredity pattern is altered.[33]

How should we interpret these results? We know that there are several biological human types, largely determined by the physical structure we inherit. It is thought that there are some hereditary factors, probably of a chemical nature, which, while giving the child its individual temperament, also provoke its birth at a time that corresponds to a specific state of the cosmos. Thus a child's birth hour would be, to a certain extent, a helpful indication of his eventual body type. This could provide the scientific basis for cosmic anthropology, which appears destined to replace the astrological

33. M. Gauquelin, *L'Hérédité planétaire* (Florence: Editions Planète, 1966).

beliefs propounded for centuries by charlatans and uneducated persons. Genetics, a rapidly expanding branch of science, could gain a new dimension, a cosmic dimension of extreme importance in this era of space travel.

Actions Unknown Until Recently

We now know that the nearest planets—Venus, Mars, Jupiter, and Saturn—are not silent bodies. In addition to their visible light they send us other messages. A radio-astronomer, J. A. Roberts, noted in 1963 that these planets, Jupiter in particular, emit powerful radio waves that have been picked up by large radio telescopes. Occasionally the "jumps" recorded by registering devices exceed those caused by the sun. Riccardi reported this as early as 1959. "Sometimes the static noises heard on the radio are not caused by interference from a nearby electrical appliance or by atmospheric phenomena but by electromagnetic waves generated by severe storms occurring in the atmosphere of Jupiter or Venus." [34]

Even more recently artificial satellites have revealed that the moon and other planets leave a wake behind them, a magnetospheric trail that causes perturbations in the solar field. In 1964 astrophysicists A. J. Dessler and E. G. Bowen calculated that the earth's magnetospheric trail is at least twenty times the distance between the earth and the sun. The magnetospheric trails of the moon and planets extend just as far into space. There must surely be a complex interaction between these wakes in the solar field. Scientists are now beginning to glimpse the disruptive role these trails could exercise on terrestrial magnetism and consequently on us. It was reported at the Fourth International Congress of

34. G. Piccardi, *Phénomènes astrophysiques et événements terrestres,* Convention at the Palais de la Découverte, January 24, 1959, p. 9.

Biometeorology that the effect of planetary heredity is influenced by the disruption of terrestrial magnetism. The effect is twice as marked on agitated days as on calm days. This fact suggests that this planetary effect depends on solar phenomena, since they are closely related to geomagnetic disturbances.[35] Therefore lunar and planetary influences on biological phenomena could conceivably be observed.

Piccardi's Explanation

But one important question remains unanswered. How does it happen that so many of our physiological reactions are subject to the effects of extraterrestrial forces? Until now only facts have been noted, and they require an explanation. A beginning has been made by G. Piccardi, Director of the Institute of Physical Chemistry at the University of Florence.

First of all, Piccardi managed to solve an old chemical mystery. An identical chemical reaction, prepared under uniform conditions, does not always occur at the same speed. It used to be thought that chance alone was responsible for these variations, but this has been disproved. By putting a metal screen over the test tubes, Piccardi found that he no longer obtained variable results. Since a metal screen blocks the disturbing agent he concluded that it must come from space. Years of daily research have revealed to Piccardi the multiple facets of this disruptive force. He has found an infinite number of cosmic influences acting on living matter in test tubes: solar activity, phasic lunar influences, and probably the influence of large planets too. He discovered an even greater influence than scientists had dared to consider—the galaxy itself.

35. M. and F. Gauquelin, *A Possible Hereditary Effect on Time of Birth in Relation With the Diurnal Movement of the Moon and the Nearest Planets*, Fourth International Biometeorological Congress, U.S.A., August 28, 1966.

While revolving about the sun, our globe is drawn across the galaxy by the sun at a speed of twelve miles per second. Its trajectory across the universe does not form a straight line. It takes the form of a helix, a sort of corkscrew. Thus the earth changes position in relationship to the galaxy's fields of force. This explains why the speed of chemical reactions varies with the months of the year. In the month of March the earth meets the fields of galactic force head-on. But in September its trajectory is parallel to these fields of force.[36]

The Liquid Necessary for Life

Vast, undreamed horizons are opening because Piccardi's discoveries are not limited to chemistry: medicine, biology, and psychology are all involved. The human body contains the same elements found in Piccardi's test tubes. Above all the human body contains water, earth's most abundant liquid and the liquid vital for life. The body is composed of 60 percent water, found in the blood, in body fluids, and in all the organs.

This liquid appears simple, but it is not. It has unusual properties. It has a pyramidic structure composed of hydrogen and oxygen atoms linked by fragile bonds that can be broken by the least external influence. Chemists like the Englishman Bernal and the American Franck have proved that at a temperature of 98.6°F, which is normal body temperature, water is in its most fragile state. In our bodies water can lose its structure extraordinarily easily under the influences emanating from the space that surrounds us. These influences may come from radiation, particles, magnetism, or gravitation.

36. G. Piccardi, *The Chemical Basis of Medical Climatology* (Springfield, Illinois: Thomas Books, 1963).

Piccardi's cosmic chemistry provides an explanation for the malaise experienced by our bodies as the result of cosmic forces that cause blood changes, modifications of body fluids, etc. Thus the scientific study of cosmic influences on our health is establishing itself as a new science, and it is searching for theories to explain these influences.

No doubt, as with every developing science, cosmic medicine will pose more questions than it can answer. Obviously we cannot hope to cite cosmic influences to explain all the fluctuations of our state of health. But certain facts are accumulating that force biologists and doctors to take this new dimension of man into consideration.

CONCLUSION:
THERAPEUTIC INDICATIONS

The domain of modern biometeorology is constantly expanding. The outline presented here is only illustration, but it does reflect this development.

The fundamental aim of researchers who have performed the experiments referred to in this work is to aid medical practitioners in relieving and treating disorders caused by atmospheric and cosmic factors. This vast undertaking is still in the embryonic stage. Biometeorological science is a discipline too new for uncontroversial therapeutics to have been developed and to have weathered the charges of critics and of time. That is why I refer only to therapeutic "indications," which are valuable and will no doubt be followed by many others.

Health and Weather Forecasts

Weather forecasting by meteorologists is our first hope. The general public and medical organizations can be informed by radio and television of any likely meteorological changes or solar eruptions to be expected in the next day or two. Together with the daily weather forecast there could be an announcement drafted by a physician advising susceptible people of the possible dangers and recommending necessary preventive measures to be taken when severe atmospheric disruptions arrive.

A similar method has been used successfully for a long time in aviation, in commercial shipping, and by the navy. But, asked de Rudder, would such a practice risk creating and maintaining in the population a veritable "weather psychosis"? We know that dangers caused by the weather do not occur only while the menacing atmospheric phenomena are passing. They can precede them, as is the case with approaching fronts, or they can follow them, as, for example, when fog concentrates noxious gases over cities.

Cardiac patients and people with high blood pressure in particular would be kept in a constant state of anxiety. So the remedy could be worse than the danger it seeks to avoid. After all, not everyone has an "anti-weather" shelter in his back yard, where he can take refuge from intense atmospheric disturbances.

Gradual education of the public would be necessary before making daily reports of potential weather dangers. Sudden traumatic announcements should always be avoided. In short, it seems that it will depend more on doctors than on their patients to watch for possible ill effects from the weather. The physician will have to remember that treatments do not have the same effectiveness under all atmospheric conditions, that patients who have undergone surgery require special attention whenever the weather is changing, and that the days following solar eruptions are especially dangerous for cardiac and tuberculous patients. In all of these cases he should take the necessary precautionary measures.

Seasonal Prophylaxis

Can we counteract the ill effects of the seasons? Most diseases show very marked seasonal variations. Medicine's role is to moderate a disease where possible in the months when it is the most dangerous and to reduce its effects to a normal level during any period of remission. This implies a sort of seasonal prophylaxis.

Supplementary amounts of vitamin D are extremely important in winter in climates where there is little sun. Both children and adults should receive them through winter until spring. For patients who are particularly threatened by the cold season, some excellent treatments have been discovered, such as cortisone for rheumatism and anticoagulants to prevent myocardial infarctions.

Vaccines are obviously the best remedy to fight the annual periodic recurrence of epidemic diseases. For maximum protection, it is advised that they be given just before the time of year when the disease strikes most severely.

Benefits from Changes of Climate

Some people are unusually sensitive to the climate of their country. Extreme weather sensitivity is the cause of almost all climatic indispositions. The doctor's first task is to combat these indispositions by "desensitizing" the patient. How? By applying the motto: "Divide and conquer." The ill urban dweller, for example, constantly experiences a large number of irritating stresses. The miasma of gas fumes, bacteria, and dust abounding in cities combines with purely climatic factors (fog, abnormal ionization, etc.) to cause his malaise. The doctor should try to counteract each of these irritating stresses individually and to alleviate their effects one by one.

The best remedy for climatic incompatibility is undeniably a "change of air," which means, quite simply, a change of climate. This change can last a few months or a few years, or may even be permanent.

A city dweller suffering from chronic asthma can be sent to a mountainous region free of infectious bacteria or irritating dust in the air. The physiological source of his complaint will be removed, and treatment will be easier in a more beneficial climate.

But the patient's return to the city remains a problem. If he is really cured, his body should be able to tolerate the previously intolerable atmospheric conditions. But there are some allergies specific to our cities that cannot be cured. In this case the only possible treatment is *permanent relocation* in a favorable climate.

Any therapy that involves sending the patient away for a change of climate should take into consideration both his temperament and the nature of his illness. There are some contraindications to this therapy. A patient whose disease is in an evolutional phase or an elderly person whose body is too exhausted should not be moved.

The locality chosen for the treatment depends partly on a suitable type of climate and partly on the nature of the illness to be treated. In mountainous areas the subject's appetite increases, he sleeps better, becomes stronger and less easily fatigued. Sea air initially creates a certain nervous overstimulation. The moderating climates of the open sea, lakes, plains, and forests also have their own special advantages.

Geographical and geological aspects should be examined carefully in every case. The doctor should check on the heat, cold, humidity, winds, and type of countryside before sending his patient away for treatment. If he has a neurasthenic patient suffering from claustrophobia, he should not choose a heavily wooded or mountainous area surrounded by high peaks blocking the horizon; the patient's psychological impression of being shut in could ruin any benefits from the change of climate. Healing usually occurs gradually through changes in the patient's endocrine system and autonomic nervous system brought about by the favorable action of the new climatic factors. Changes of climate are often associated with climatic health resorts, whose beneficial properties have been recognized since ancient times. Describing climatic health resorts (spas) could fill an entire book. I am only mentioning them briefly because their study is beyond the field of biometeorology. However, here are details of two modern therapies linked with climate: heliotherapy and thalassotherapy.

Heliotherapy is based on the curative and bactericidal properties of the sun's rays. Depending on the disease, different types of heliotherapy are recommended, and the patient may be sent to mountains, plains, or the seashore. Generally speaking, this treatment is helpful to patients suffering from tuberculosis and bronchitis and to persons afflicted with infectious skin diseases. But there are some contraindications. Cardiac patients and people with high blood pressure should not be treated with intensive heliotherapy.

Thalassotherapy consists in utilizing the beneficial effects of the sea climate with its abundance of ozone, iodine, magnesium, and sodium in the air, and the curative properties of sea baths. The patient can swim in either the ocean or special salt-water pools. Other therapies can be added: sea-mud baths, sand baths, and seaweed baths. Thalassotherapy is a sort of "salt water" health cure. It is an excellent treatment for rheumatism and for some climatically induced glandular malfunctions that have resisted other treatments. Extremely nervous patients are also favorably affected by sea climate. In the opinion of Dr. Haberlin, the results of this treatment vary according to the type of nervous complaint. The treatment is generally contraindicated for tuberculous, asthmatic, and cardiac patients.

Artificial Climatotherapy

Patients who for professional, economic, or family reasons cannot or do not wish to leave their place of residence can now benefit from new climatological therapeutics developed by medical science, such as pharmaceutical remedies, artificial aero-ionization, aerosol treatments, and climatic chambers.

Dr. Assmann wrote that it is the people with poor autonomic-nervous-system regulation who suffer especially from the weather. Their disorders are often aggravated by the exhausting life of modern man. Medicine has developed various pharmaceutical products to combat the harmful effects of atmospheric conditions on the nervous system. These are called "sympatholytic" or "parasympatholytic" agents. The nature of the disease being treated determines which kind should be used. Obviously, different temperaments require different medications.

Respiratory enzymes are included in this type of remedy. They were mentioned previously in reference to high-altitude sickness because they improve the respiration of those people who cannot tolerate oxygen rarefaction.

The disadvantage of these medications lies in the fact that the patient quickly becomes accustomed to them. Their effectiveness diminishes considerably, and a change of climate may ultimately become necessary.

The clinical effects of aero-ionization are numerous and have been studied extensively. In the USSR atmospheric ionization is a very popular treatment for a large number of diseases, especially asthma and rheumatic disease. In the United States it has been used successfully to relieve the allergic symptoms from ragweed, which causes severe hay fever.

Many hospitals have now installed ionized-air generators.

These are very intricate machines because we must have absolute control over the percentage of positive and negative ions disseminated into the air. Negative ions with their tonic yet relaxing properties are more often recommended than positive ions, which are stimulating and irritating.

Aerosol treatment consists of spraying the recommended curative medicament into the air in fine particles, liquid or solid. These particles become charged with electricity as a result of their violent friction with the atmosphere on dispersion. This property allows them to penetrate deep into the patient's respiratory tract, where they remain once their electrical charge is lost. Aerosol treatments have important clinical applications. They are used primarily in treating diseases of the respiratory tract of atmospheric origin. Sinusitis, an inflammation of the sinuses, can be treated with an antibiotic spray, as can chronic laryngitis. In some countries sprays containing spasmolytic agents are used to treat bronchial asthma. They are even more effective when applied in a climatic chamber.

Climatic chambers are the latest major form of artificial climatotherapy, and health specialists hope for very successful results from them. A climatic chamber is a hermetically sealed room where one or more specific climatic factors can be reproduced and controlled artificially. It has been used for experimentation on thermoregulation and on the body's ability to adapt to various climatic stresses. But it was created above all for therapeutic purposes.

The patient in a climatic chamber finds himself in surroundings necessary for the improvement of his health without having to leave his residence. Obviously, it is almost impossible to modify satisfactorily *all* the elements of a given climate at the same time. The factors now being controlled are air temperature, humidity, oxygen pressure, ultraviolet rays, and ionization.

Here is an illustration of the advantages of artificial climatic isolation of patients. In a French hospital center some excellent results have been obtained using a low-pressure chamber over the past several years with cases of sinusitis resisting all other treatments. The oxygen pressure of the climatic chamber is altered to create high-altitude atmospheric conditions. The air is purified and maintained at a constant level of humidity. In addition, infrared and ultraviolet rays are also provided. In a very short time the patient feels as though he is on top of a high mountain with no discomfort other than mild shortness of breath and a slight buzzing in the ears. These discomforts are amply compensated for by the effectiveness of the treatment. The most persistent sinusitis can be conquered in about fifteen one-hour therapy sessions.

The Future of Biometeorology

The possible applications of biometeorology are only beginning to unfold. Aided by technical means and ample materials, we may well be able to modify climates considerably, making them more favorable. Man is not yet able to transform the whole planet, which is just as well. But what is worthwhile is that he can improve the atrocious climates of large cities. It is imperative that medical prophylaxis be combined with meaningful city planning. It is imperative that urban specialists hear the cries of biometeorologists and take notice of the scientific discoveries of this new discipline. Our health and that of our children depends on action from those responsible for protecting us from the many dangers pointed out throughout this work.

Every year biometeorology gains more followers. More scientists are becoming interested in this field, are collecting more knowledge, and imparting their discoveries at conferences which receive more and more publicity. Both prudence and audacity are needed in such a complex field. Researchers must not forget the wise advice handed down centuries ago by Hippocrates:

"Life is short and the art is long; the occasion fleeting; experience fallacious and judgment difficult. The physician must not only be prepared to do what is right himself but also to make the patient, the attendants, and externals cooperate."

APPENDIX

I. *INFLUENCE OF SEASON ON NORMAL PHYSIOLOGICAL PROCESSES*

Physiological Processes	Observed Seasonal Changes
Blood pressure	Higher in winter from October to March
Calcium and phosphate in the blood	Minimum February–March, maximum in August
Blood volume	Lower in winter than in summer
Total blood protein, albumin, hemoglobin	Often higher in winter than in summer
Leukocytes	Maximum around December, minimum in August
Blood-sedimentation rate	Greater in winter than in summer
Bleeding after treatment with anticoagulants	Maximum January–February, minimum in July
Capillary fragility	Highest fragility from January to April, low from July to December; high fragility probably due to vitamin P deficiency in winter

Physiological Processes	Observed Seasonal Changes
General metabolism	Maximum in summer, minimum in winter
Thyroid activity	Maximum in winter, minimum in summer
Gastro-acidity	Hyperacidity high in winter, low in summer
Gastro-alkalinity	High in summer, low in winter
Growth of children	Slow growth in winter, rapidly increasing in spring
Birth weight	Newborn babies: greatest June–July, smallest December–March
Birth frequency	Highest number of conceptions in June (legitimate children) or May (illegitimate); stillborn maximum in January
Mortality	In W. Europe maximum December–February, minimum July–August

(Extracts taken from S. W. Tromp, *Medical Biometeorology*, Elsevier, 1963, Table 39, p. 575.)

II. INFLUENCE OF SEASON ON PATHOLOGICAL PROCESSES

Non-infectious Diseases

Arteriosclerotic heart disease and apoplexy	Maximum January–February, minimum July–August
Bronchitis	Maximum in winter, low in spring and summer
Bronchial asthma	Maximum August–November

Physiological Processes	Observed Seasonal Changes
Peptic ulcer	Maximum December–February, minimum in June
Duodenal ulcer	Maximum May and November (only in males)
Appendicitis	Usually more common in warm summers
Glaucoma	High in winter (maximum in November), low in summer
Rheumatic diseases	Usually more common during the cold, humid, windy seasons
Diabetes	Coma more common in winter
Goiter (exophthalmic)	Maximum in May, minimum in summer
Mental diseases	Maximum unrest in spring; birth frequency of schizophrenics most common January–March; more anencephalics born in December
Suicide	Maximum in spring, minimum in winter
Hay fever	Usually May–June
Rickets	Most frequent in winter due to vitamin D deficiency; minimum July–August

Infectious Diseases

Tuberculosis	Mortality increases in spring, and so does sensitivity to tuberculin test
Scarlatina	Maximum in October

Physiological Processes	Observed Seasonal Changes
Diphtheria	Maximum in November, increasing from August
Influenza	Maximum from December to February, increasing from September
Pneumonia	Maximum from December to February
Cerebrospinal meningitis	Maximum from December to April, minimum in August
Variola	Maximum in March, increasing from September
Conjunctivitis	Maximum in July
Cholera	Increasing from May to September, maximum in August
Typhoid fever	Maximum in August, increasing from May to September
Poliomyelitis	Maximum August–September, increasing from May to September
Bacillary dysentery	Maximum in summer, increasing from May to September

(Extracts taken from S. W. Tromp, *Medical Biometeorology*, Elsevier, 1963, Table 39, p. 579 .)

REFERENCES

ASSMANN, D., *Die Wetterfühligkeit des Menschen* (Jena: Fischer, 1963)

BERG, H., *Solar-terrestrische Beziehungen in Meteorologie und Biologie* (Leipzig: Geest und Portig, 1957)

CARLES, L. M., *Agents pathogènes et climat* (Masson, 1945)

DUHOT, E., *Les climats et l'organisme humain* (P.U.F., 1951)

DUHOT, E., and FONTAN, M., *Le Thermalisme* (P.U.F., 1963)

GAUQUELIN, M., *L'hérédité planétaire* (Planète, 1966)

I.N.S.E.E., *Etudes statistiques,* Publication périodique

INSTITUT NATIONAL D'ETUDES DEMOGRAPHIQUES, *Population,* Revue trimestrielle

INSTITUT NATIONAL D'HYGIENE, Bulletin périodique

JOLY, R., *Hippocrate et la médecine grecque* (N.R.F. [Idees], 1964)

MISSEMARD, A., *L'homme et le climat* (Plon, 1937)

PETERSEN, W. F., *The Patient and the Weather,* I-IV, (Chicago, 1935)

PICCARDI, G., *The Chemical Basis of Medical Climatology* (Springfield: Thomas Books, 1963)

PIERY, M., MILHAUD, M., and VAN DER ELST, R., *Traité de climatologie biologique et médicale* (Masson, 1934)

REINBERG, A., and GHATA, J., *Rythmes et cycles biologiques* (P.U.F., 1937)

RIVOLIER, J., *La biométéorologie* (Diagrammes, No. 95, 1964)

DE RUDDER, B., *Grundriss einer Meteorobiologie des Menschen* (Berlin: Springer, 1952)

SCHAEFER, K. E., *Man's Dependence on the Earthly Atmosphere* (New York: Macmillan, 1958)

Symposium International sur les relations entre phénomènes solaires et terrestres en chimie physique et en biologie (Brussels: Presses Académiques Européennes, 1960)

TROMP, S. W., *Medical Biometeorology* (New York: Elsevier, 1963)

VIAUT, A., *La Météorologie* (P.U.F., 1963)

Zemlia vo Vseliennoi, collective work (Moscow: State Editions, 1964)

Specialized Works

The reader who wishes to pursue his interest in a particular topic should refer to the various scientific works mentioned in the course of this work.